An Insider's Guide to
HOME
HEALTH
CARE

An Insider's Guide to
HOME HEALTH CARE

Tova Navarra, BA, RN

Margaret Lundrigan Ferrer, MSW, LCSW

SLACK Incorporated, 6900 Grove Road, Thorofare, NJ 08086

Publisher: John H. Bond
Editorial Director: Amy E. Drummond

Printed in the United States of America

Navarra, Tova.
        An insider's guide to home health care / Tova Navarra, Margaret
        Lundrigan Ferrer.
             p.   cm.
        Includes bibliographic references
        ISBN 1-55642-287-3 (alk. paper)
1. Home care services. I. Ferrer, Margaret Lundrigan. II. Title.
[DNLM: 1. Home Care Services. 2. Caregivers--psychology. WY 115 N321i
1996]
RA645.3.N38   1996
362.1'4--dc20
DNLM/DLC   96-31957
for Library of Congress   CIP

Published by: SLACK Incorporated
                   6900 Grove Road
                   Thorofare, NJ 08086 USA
                   Telephone 609-848-1000   Fax 609-853-5991

Dedication

To Rose Lane Leslie, my grandmother, who even after her transition has never failed to love and help me.
TN

I dedicate this book to my mother, Margaret M. Lundrigan, who showed me all the important things in life: children, books, gardens, and most of all, love and friendship.
MLF

Both authors also wish to extend a special dedication of this work to Marcia Granucci, a New Jersey registered nurse and mother of two teenagers, who gave her life at age 45, as she made a home visit last November. Ms. Granucci's patient had murdered his elderly parents and then shot her as she entered his home. The home-care community suffers her loss and will always be reminded that caregivers' risks are never small for the sake of their patients.

Contents

Acknowledgments

The authors wish to thank those who supported the making of this book by contributing their enthusiasm, knowledge, literary insights, references and research materials, interviews, editorial services and compassion: John Bond, Publisher, and Amy Drummond, Editorial Director, at SLACK Inc.; Val J. Halamandaris, president, and Margo Gillman, of the National Association for Home Care (NAHC), Washington, D.C.; Robert A. Fusco, president, Nancy Tait and David Fluhrer, of Olsten Kimberly National Resource Center; Mark Kator, CEO and president of Coler Memorial Hospital, New York; Mary Lou Galantino, assistant professor of physical therapy at The Richard Stockton College of New Jersey; Dr. Bella May, Professor of PT at the Medical College of Georgia; Joan Powers, MSW, LCSW, of the VNA of Central Jersey; Teresa Vaccaro, RN; Cary Katz, MA, education consultant; Ann Healy, manager of the Home Health Aide department of the VNA of Central Jersey; Carolyn B. Smith, president of Eden Home Care Services, Inc.; Rose Treihart, RN, MA; Gloria Coppola, director of the Garden State Center for Holistic Health Care, Lakewood; Mary Brasseur, who calls herself "the tarnished mystic"; David M. Campbell, Tracy Sander, Jennifer J. Cahill, and Debra Clarke, all of SLACK Inc.; Rafael Conde of Media Resource Services, New York City; Joan Hermann, MSW, ACSW, at Fox Chase Cancer Center, Philadelphia, Pa.; nutritionist Mary Burgess; our good friend Irene ("Fiona") Haran, and our children, Meghan and Brendan Ferrer and Yolanda, Johnny and Mitzi Navarra and Guy Fleming — truly significant others who teach us something new every day.

About the Authors

Tova Navarra, BA, RN, is a magna cum laude graduate of Seton Hall University, a registered nurse, former contributing editor of the *American Journal of Nursing,* syndicated health columnist for Copley News Service (based in San Diego, Ca.), and the author of 13 books, including *Wisdom for Caregivers*; *On My Own: Helping Kids Help Themselves*; *Therapeutic Communication*; *Allergies A-Z*; *The Encyclopedia of Vitamins, Minerals and Supplements*; *Your Body: Highlights of Human Anatomy*; *Howell and Farmingdale: A Social and Cultural History*; and *The New Jersey Shore: A Vanishing Splendor.* She has had articles published in The New York Times and many other newspapers and journals. Also a former feature writer and art critic for the Asbury Park Press and the mother of two grown children, Ms. Navarra is working on several new books for adults and children. She lives in Monmouth County, New Jersey, with her husband, John, her shih tzu, Francis, and two highly opinionated rabbits.

Margaret Lundrigan Ferrer, MSW, LCSW, is a Pace University and Rutgers University alumna who has worked as supervisor of grant research for the Visiting Nurse Association of Central Jersey and as an oncology/hospice social worker at Riverview Medical Center in Red Bank, New Jersey. With an additional background in drug and alcohol counseling, Ms. Ferrer is a freelance writer who has had articles on professional boundaries published in *Cancer Practice* and The Two River Times. An historian by avocation, she has written *Richmond Town and Lighthouse Hill* and co-authored *Levittown,* two of Arcadia's *Images of America* book series. She is also a certified school social worker and member of a child-study team. She lives in Monmouth County with her husband, John, two children, Meghan, 15, and Brendan, 11, two English bulldogs, and a cockatiel who likes her best.

Preface

The Chinese word for "crisis" consists of two characters: one meaning danger and the other meaning opportunity. When an author undertakes the writing of a book on home health care — a book such as this with a hearty intent of sending information (some of which may be strong, unattractive stuff that goes with the health caregiving territory) and encouragement for survival and self-actualized growth — she is definitely confronting a crisis.

The "danger" may be manifold. The first lion to pass is the one roaring, "You will not please everyone." Although anxiety comes of the realization that there are so many concepts, philosophies, experiences and examples that an author simply cannot represent all places and ideas, it is assuaged somewhat by the laws that no one knows everything and there's no fool you can't learn from.

The second danger lies in risking. An author takes many risks when she decides to tell some lovely as well as some awful truths about home health care as an industry. But, at very least, the risk should yield a better prepared caregiver and a better cared-for patient. In this book, we have chosen to use the terms "patient" and "client" interchangeably because both are appropriate.

Accordingly, we use "care provider," "health professional," "caregiver," and other similar terms interchangeably. Each health care discipline chooses its vocabulary for good reasons, and we do respect that. In addition, we provide a glossary of terms in hopes of bridging jargon gaps among health disciplines. Communication, after all, stands at the helm of all care, from the most intricate neurosurgery to the unembellished patting of a patient's hand.

Our desire, and thus our "opportunity," is that caregivers will feel enriched by this book and, by also using it as an orientation "primer" in workshops and other training programs, transfer that enrichment to their colleagues, their patients and, in fact, all human beings. Please feel free to write to us in care of SLACK Inc., to enrich our perspectives. Whether at the bedside or the computer, we make sincere efforts toward mutual understanding and sharing as part of the health care system, and, it is hoped, as an example for its growth.

Foreword

At the beginning of this century, it was common to receive care in the home and to have your physician visit you there. Now, as the 21st century approaches, we find ourselves returning to the home and to a health care model based on the values of community-based care. This is comforting. For while institutional care over the past decades brought us many medical wonders, it also brought us an increasingly depersonalized health care delivery system and a health care infrastructure that our nation cannot afford to support.

This "renaissance" in home care is the result, I believe, of many divergent trends coming together at one point in time: the availability of sophisticated medical technology that has made it safe and convenient to administer a wide range of therapies in the home; a growing aged population and thus, growing demand; pressure from managed care organizations and federal and state governments to contain costs; a consumer ground swell in favor of home- and community-based care, which allows people to receive treatment in the privacy of their own homes with the support of the family and loved ones; and the simple economic fact that home care today provides the same quality care once only available in institutions—but for far less. According to the National Association for Home Care, the cost for one day of home care in 1994 averaged $83, compared to $1,756 for one day in the hospital.

The renaissance in home health care is also being fueled by the industry's own transformation from what was merely an add-on service to institutional care, into a huge industry of its own. In 1994, home health care represented only 2% to 3% of health care expenditures. By the year 2000, it is projected that it will account for about 10%. Over the next few years, then, our homes will become a primary site of care. To prepare for this, home health care companies will need to increase their economies of scale and scope. Size is important because it will allow providers to keep costs down while they deliver care to increasingly larger geographic networks. Scope is necessary because managed care organizations are demanding the integrated and seamless delivery of services. This means nursing services, infusion services, home medical equipment and respiratory therapy services will be provided by "network" managers with the resources to coordinate all aspects of care.

The benefit of MCOs is simpler administration, elimination of redundant care, and lower costs. For patients the benefit is truly coordinated care. As part of this transformation, home health care must also continue to develop standards of care utilizing the best industry practices. Quality guidelines as established by JCAHO and the NCQA must be adhered to across the board and become the industry norm. And care should be outcome-driven, based on critical pathways or care protocols. This will ensure our patients receive only the best and most appropriate care.

The expanded use of information systems and more sophisticated data collection will also be necessary as we provide more care for patient populations. Increasingly, home health care is being asked to provide care for chronic conditions such as asthma, diabetes and heart disease. Home care programs that educate patients and teach them to manage their condition have already proven to be successful, with patients greatly benefiting from an improved quality of life. And the overall health care system benefits too, because costs for care of the disease are reduced not once or twice, but over entire lifetimes.

At the same time as we undergo this transformation, there will be an increased need for management sophistication within the industry. As we are asked to manage more aspects of a patient's care, home health care will need the expertise of managers who are generalists as well as specialists. The industry, until recently, was fragmented into nursing, infusion, and home medical equipment. The demand of seamless care is driving integration and consolidation of these areas. The result is we will need managers with experience in all aspects of home care, who can provide the vision and leadership to help create tomorrow's new health care delivery system. In addition, as this system is created, we will see the role of nurses and other caregiver professionals enlarged. They will become the gatekeepers for home care, working with physicians and drawing on a wide range of community resources to provide a "circle of care."

We will also see an increased need for developing relationships with physicians. This group is generally unfamiliar with home care and its benefits. Working with them, we can increase their knowledge base of the benefits home care provides their patients.

Finally, I believe we will see a growing role in the influence and importance of consumers in health care. This is already happening in some of the most advanced managed care markets like Minnesota. There, health care coalitions are looking to restore choice to consumers. A more active consumer would portend well for home health care's growth. It also means now is the time for our industry to become customer-focused and service-oriented. Those home health operations which embrace continuous quality improvement today will be the ones which flourish tomorrow.

This is a great time for the home health care industry. We are in a position to help create a health care delivery system that in a sense brings people back to the future. The natural setting of the home is the best place to provide holistic care, which considers a patient's emotional and spiritual, as well as physical, needs. It is where patients overwhelmingly prefer to be cared for. And it is affordable, which means it can continue to meet growing future demand. I feel very lucky to be a part of this industry at this point in its history. Now it's up to all of us to contribute to its writing so we can be proud of the job we do.

Robert A. Fusco, President
Olsten Kimberly QualityCare

Introduction

"There's no place like home."
Dorothy in "The Wizard of Oz"

"Home Sweet Home": the place in which we eat, sleep, relax, entertain, work, play, think, and share with a spouse, a friend, a pet, or not with anyone. That unique place that may be dark and confining or where sunlight comes in through the windows full and warm. A room or a suite of rooms filled with one's personality and memories and spirit, whether decorated to the hilt or sparsely furnished. Home is a mansion on a hill, a Cape Cod house in a suburban development, a city apartment, a tiny segment of a communal dwelling, a shack by the sea. For some, home means a room in a motel designated for the homeless or a refrigerator box in an alley.

Despite its character, home is where all health care began. The first caregivers were the people closest to the patient — a term derived from the Greek word *pema*, which means suffering. Perhaps a doctor, "medicine man," or local healer was called in. Midwives or untrained but experienced women delivered babies. The aged were cared for by their kin. Neighbors helped out when they could. Essentially, people took care of each other no matter what physical or mental deficits presented themselves. The hospital, if available at all, was reserved for extreme cases.

Societal evolution established the practice of sending the ill out of their homes for care, such as tuberculosis victims leaving for lengthy stays in sanitariums. Patients went back to their homes if they recovered. Now, ironically, after we've been a culture that has built medical centers, rehabilitation hospitals and other imposing health care organizations and watched them grow monstrously large, health care is turning back into an intimate, personalized process that takes place in the patient's home.

About 20 years ago, almost all of the patients sent home from the hospital in medical danger or still in need of great amounts of care were the terminally ill for whom nothing more could be done. To them, daily maintenance and palliative care were all that could be offered. This created a filtered form of the hospice movement that emerged during the Crusades, when a hospice was an actual place of refuge, not a program supervised by an agency or health facility, as it typically is today. Private-duty nurses, therapists, home health aides, nurse's aides, social workers and other caregivers traveled to the patient's residence to bathe, feed, medicate and support whatever life the patient had left.

Introduction

Like the legendary country doctors who often accepted a pig, fresh eggs or garden vegetables as payment, modern caregivers perform their services on the patient's turf. Instead of being authority figures employed by an institution with its unique culture, home health caregivers must cope with whatever circumstances prevail.

The first mission of this book is to inform — and thereby empower — professional and non-professional home health caregivers before they knock on someone's door and find unexpected difficulties or horrors within that dwelling. Health care, like the universe, is a "field of all possibilities," as endocrinologist and author Dr. Deepak Chopra put it. The possibilities are infinite for both the caregiver and the patient. One episode of "Seinfeld," a popular television situation-comedy, made this point surprisingly well. Elaine, Seinfeld's girlfriend on the show, volunteers to make home visits for a health care agency. Jerry Seinfeld and his pal, George, also volunteer. The patients are senior citizens who need companionship.

Elaine's first visit is to an interesting, pleasant woman who has a goiter the size of a football protruding from her neck. Taken aback, Elaine feels so uncomfortable that she has trouble making eye contact with the woman, much less good conversation. She later complains to Jerry that she was not given any "goiter information" by the agency, and it was an unnerving experience not to have known about it in advance.

Jerry's patient turned out to be a crotchety old man who teased Jerry viciously, barking, "Wanna change my diaper?" The man then told Jerry to "get the hell out of my house." George's patient was a nice man who "fired" George because he couldn't stand his cynical outlook on life. If this is situation comedy — and it was a funny show — can you imagine how caregivers in the real world must feel when similar situations arise for them? Not clever, not funny. Home care is serious and the caregiver is accountable.

Health caregivers — physician, registered nurse, practical nurse, nurse practitioner, social worker, physical therapist, occupational therapist, their assistants (PTAs and OTAs), speech therapist, respiratory therapist, nurse's aide, home health aide, homemaker, chore person, volunteer, massage therapist, companion and spiritual counselor or clergy — now create their own select health care team, with most patients directing and participating in their care. The "institution" exists only in the sense that the team members work together to mobilize a specific set of services and interact with the patient and significant others in an efficient, professional manner. While the medical center or other facility stands in the background as an option for treatment, the health team's joint workplace is their patient's domain.

Because of this division of authority and ethics that embrace both patients' and caregivers' rights, difficulties abound. Home care may well seem a petri dish of potential problems that can ambush an unsuspecting caregiver. Here we hope to augment a caregiver's training and effectiveness by recounting memorable, anecdotal vignettes citing patient/caregiver situations. Through both the successful and difficult experiences of others, caregivers may add to their knowledge, experience base and critical thinking. The ideal result is better care for the patient and a strengthening, rather than depletion, of the ability of the home caregiver team.

The second mission centers on teaching each team member who the other members are and what they're doing. Roles and duties are defined. We also point out how some roles can overlap, which may cause tension, competitiveness and confusion in home care. The fact that significant others entwine themselves in the health-care team may also complicate things, when instead it can facilitate optimal care, including care the team members themselves require to keep going and to cooperate with each other.

A good part of self-care involves an understanding of "the big picture." The chapter on the history of home health care renews our motivation, values and quests in American society. "The Fine Tradition" of home care deserves a fresh perspective in terms of how caregivers maneuver their way through medical, bureaucratic, ethical and personal processes. Caregivers also need to know the communities in which they work; the community, after all, is where the patient is.

For example, does a community offer valuable resources to families involved with home care of a loved one? Is there a support system to be found in neighbors, police, teachers, township administrators, religious groups, merchants, etc.? How safe are the surroundings? These are some of the questions that arise when a caregiver finds herself in sole charge of a totally incapacitated patient who lives in a large, intimidatingly creaky house in an isolated area. Or when a caregiver spends eight hours or more in an overcrowded, poorly maintained apartment building in a high-crime neighborhood.

Even a caregiver assigned to a lavish home in an affluent town has concerns. Will a costly object break accidentally or disappear during a caregiver's visit? Will servants and groundskeepers interfere with the caregivers' comings and goings? Will a caregiver harbor some resentment toward the patient and his family because of their wealth, or simply be uncomfortable in such an environment? To our knowledge, most home health training focuses on duties, procedures, treatments and other hands-on services, basic communication and role boundaries, and identifying the patient's needs and how to meet them.

Introduction

It seems important, then, to address the myriad situations — from the physical environment to the emotional gamut of human interaction — not typically part of formal training. That medical students have only recently begun to study the mind/body connection and the value of getting on a "feeling level" with patients illustrates an interesting point. For many years, whatever bedside manner a doctor employed was accepted by a good number of patients. If he or she were brusque and unsmiling, it rarely occurred to a patient to seek a more approachable physician. Somehow it became ingrained in us — a population of potential patients — to set our sights on being cured or relieved of pain rather than insist on holistic care. In the hospital, patients were to be treated for their maladies. Once the patient returned home, holistic care was available because the significant others knew the patient as more than just a physical entity.

In the home, the home health caregivers can become as familiar with a patient as are the significant others. Here again, the effect of bringing health care to the home forces the caregiver-patient relationship to regroup, in a sense, from the less personal, unconditionally accepted atmosphere of the hospital to a veritable extension of significant others. In this book, we confront some of the trickier aspects of the changed relationship so caregivers can plan ahead and put their own "houses" in order.

Our third mission is to inspire home health caregivers to forge new paths in the home health field and to grow professionally and spiritually. Caregivers are not martyrs (although a few like to have their care emanate that quality). They need to know they are doing good things for people even when recognition is infrequent and meager. Home health aides, PTAs, OTAs, nurse's aides, homemakers and volunteers, for example, are often considered "workhorses" who carry out the orders of their superiors. We acknowledge the "workhorses" as health team members who have as integral a stake in the well-being and care of patients as the other caregivers. The aide, PTA, OTA or other caregiver may in fact be doing work on the assistant level as part of a professional career plan. In the case of the aide, professionalization of that role may be in order. Furthermore, a talented assistant, home health or nurse's aide deserves the opportunity to become a health professional if he or she chooses.

Opportunities must evolve through our health care delivery system. Professionals should encourage others to acquire the skills necessary to meet the mind/body needs of an increasingly diverse society. Home health agencies, medical centers and other organizations such as Reaching Up, founded by John F. Kennedy Jr., Esq., have begun to champion continuing education for the caregivers traditionally (and unfortunately) thought of as the "lower echelon."

Fortifying the caregiving ranks, we hope, will not be looked upon as creating a glut of workers and professionals, but rather as a well-received cultural force that has the power to help people heal themselves in their own homes. Then, as managed health care intensifies, the home will truly be "Home Sweet Home," the place that shelters, nurtures and heals all who go there.

Tova Navarra
Margaret Lundrigan Ferrer

Chapter 1

Home Care: A Fine Tradition

The hazards of sickness, accident, invalidism...and old age should be provided for through insurance.
Theodore Roosevelt, 1912

The healer has to keep striving for...the space...in which healer and patient can reach out to each other as travelers sharing the same broken human condition.
Henri J. M. Rouwen, *Reaching Out*

In 1897, in a tenement on the Lower East Side of Manhattan, a male infant came into the world at the hand of a midwife who proclaimed him so sickly that he would not live. He was still telling the story of his birth at age 98, six months before he died peacefully in his bed in southern California.

During her voluntary stint as a Civil War nurse, American author Louisa May Alcott contracted typhoid from unsanitary hospital conditions. Never fully recovered, Alcott later became a successful writer who recounted in *Little Women* the extensive home care and eventual death of her sister Elizabeth, who suffered complications resulting from scarlet fever. Alcott's mother and younger sister, May, also died, leaving a niece for Alcott to rear. Ultimately, Alcott suffered severe fatigue and pain and went to live with her physician, Rhoda Lawrence, until her death in 1888, at the age of 56.

This was the original nature of health care. The disabled children; the frail, perhaps senile, elderly; the mentally retarded relative; the orphan taken in by a neighborhood family; the chronically ill spouse; the woman in labor; the otherwise needy person—mostly all stayed home.

The history of health care begins with care people received at home long before there were hospitals and medical centers and physicians' offices. For many of the Baby Boom generation of the 1950s and 1960s, the idea of babies born at home and the ill and dying cared for at home evokes picturesque images of the Wild West and "Little House on the

Prairie." It is startling to realize that only about 50 years ago, non-professional midwives delivered babies, the ill were cared for at home, and most people did, in fact, die in their own beds. Rather than being the exception, home health care was the norm.

The technological revolution that continues to affect communications, transportation, agriculture, and manufacturing left an impressive mark on the field of health care. The last half-century saw remarkable advances in the field of pharmacology, such as broad-spectrum antibiotics and polio and other vaccines, the emergence of chemotherapy and radiation, renal dialysis, open-heart surgery, organ transplantation and the introduction of microscopic and laser surgery. In fewer than 100 years, surgery that had once been a prospect that almost invariably meant excruciating pain would become relatively pain-free as a result of refined anesthesia. We have witnessed the eradication of smallpox and the near-eradication of diphtheria and other diseases. We are able to treat many types of cancers successfully, and we have experienced an increase by 12 years in the average life expectancy. The amount of scientific knowledge gained in this 50-year period was not much less than that attributed to the previous 2,000 years. Now, as health professionals and scientists confront AIDS and other new diseases and a resurgence of tuberculosis and other old diseases, we go forth in the "brave new world" of medicine, art, and science we boldly entered.

As medical and health care became increasingly technological, however, the average person became less likely to be involved in his own or anyone else's care. Furthermore, people became less knowledgeable on simple primary care and more likely to turn to expert assistance. Health care had taken a turn from an emphasis on personal prevention and familial responsibility for much primary care to a far more reactive stance. Not unlike the inner-city kids who have virtually no idea how the food reaches the table, we began to see health care as something beyond the scope of the average individual. We abdicated the responsibility to the health care professional. Technology had pushed us beyond the point where strep throat could escalate into scarlet fever that threatened deafness or a slight summer chill that held the danger of emerging as the dreaded polio virus. Death was coming much closer to being an option. As English historian Alexander Toynbee once remarked, "Death is un-American."

Hospitals existed as early as the 4th century, and there is historical and scientific evidence that some early peoples, perhaps including the Mayans, performed various surgeries. But until the last century, the locus of the vast majority of medical and health care was the home. The pioneering of the American Frontier shares much with other cultures in the way in which health care was delivered. A family crossing the continent had virtually no access to professional medical care and would by necessity be forced to rely upon prevention and their own limited knowledge if illness did occur. When sickness struck, it could be swift and merciless. The plains of America were dotted with makeshift graves of children and family members who died on the arduous quest for better lives.

Immigrants coming to American shores faced even greater risks. Those who could afford only steerage accommodations typically spent 8 to 10 days in difficult conditions they were fortunate to survive. Located in the lowermost portion of the ship, passengers lacked adequate ventilation and sanitation, often suffered from sea-sickness, and were greatly overcrowded. The trip afforded the perfect conditions for the transmission and incubation of disease. Because several to many passengers died per trip, the vessels earned the name "coffin ships." Those strong and fortunate enough to survive the trip faced similar challenges as they commenced life in the New World. Those moving West encountered the dangers of intercontinental migration, including brutal extremes of sweltering heat to temperatures below freezing, lack of water and medicine, and isolation from societal supports. Those who remained in the cities dealt with nightmarish urban problems that were no less dangerous. The following excerpt from *The Slums as a Common Nuisance* by John Savage recounts the ultimate outcome of such dangers.

> "These apartments, during the summer of 1832, while the Asiatic cholera prevailed in Albany, were inhabited, as one witness stated, by between forty and fifty, and as another stated, by between sixty and eighty Irish emigrants, each apartment containing between two and three families. The premises were extremely filthy; under the floors were twenty tan vats, most of which were filled with putrid stagnant water, which oozed through the floors on walking over them. Some of the inmates were sick, and two, a woman and child lying dead in the house."

The Development of Public Health Housing

The existence of such abhorrent conditions created the need for the development of public health nursing. In response to similar conditions in England in the late 1800s and early 1900s, William Rathbone requested that his friend Florence Nightingale develop a plan for nurses to provide care in the home. Although Rathbone was too busy to become actively involved in this type of care personally, Nightingale proved herself a true visionary by developing nursing as a profession, including a plan for nursing care that came to be known as District Nursing. The concept of district nursing to provide care to poor people in their homes was quickly exported to the United States.

In 1893, American social worker Lillian D. Wald, whose name was to become synonymous with the concept of visiting nurses and the Visiting Nurse Associations of today, helped found the Henry Street Settlement House in New York City. Over the next 40 years, Wald and her nurses provided nursing visits to immigrants in the poor, overcrowded tenements of the Lower East Side. At the same time, they served as prototypes for the development of public health nursing in the United States. During those formative years, the neighborhood nurses waged a war of prevention and education against the horrendous health conditions that languished in the slums of New York.

The nurses formed a comprehensive level of practice that included case finding (seeking out residents who would benefit from nursing intervention), health care treatment, education geared to prevention and wellness, and establishing a trust and therapeutic bond with their patients. The visiting nurse grew to be a respected and trusted member of the community. In many ways, the visiting nurse was an emissary of welcome in the New World for newly arriving immigrants.

Adept at activating the patient's support system and advocating for the patient in the larger community, the nurses gained strength and validation as a positive force in American society. In *Public Health Nursing Legacy*, Joyce Zerwekh describes a case in which a Henry Street nurse was working with a paralyzed mother. The woman was lifted into a chair in the morning and had to remain there until her husband returned home from work.

> "We begged the Street Cleaning Commission to change the man's station to the blocks near the tenement home, and also to grant the privilege of the man's help at home for fifteen minutes a day....At ten thirty in the morning the nurse appeared, gave the patient her bath, made the bed, completed her toilet. She then went down the stairs and beckoned the sweeper. He lifted the woman to her chair and without delay returned to his work for the city. The household, now well organized, kept mother, father, and four children knit together in a family unit. After the day's work the sweeper returned to the home and lifted the wife back to bed; with her shortened day and better care, she was not too exhausted to give housewifely supervision to dinner preparations and the other home duties shared by husband and children."

Here the nurse not only provided medical care but also activated the natural strengths of the family and intervened with the community to facilitate the well-being of the patient and family.

Here, too, we see that the nurse did not confine her concerns to the physical health alone, but entered into social issues as well. A prime example of this type of concern is cited by Lillian Wald in which she addresses the issues of truancy and child labor: "Examination of the school attendance of children who do home work bears testimony to its relation to truancy. Josephine, 11 years of age, stays out of school to work on finishing; Francesca, age 12, to sew buttons on coats; Santa, 9 years old, to pick out nut meats; Catherine, 8 years old, sews on tags; Tiffy, another 8-year-old, helps her mother finish; Giuseppe, age 10, is a deft worker on artificial flowers."

The Development of Social Work

In a similar manner, social work efforts in America started in the home. Based on the Elizabethan Poor Law of 1601, the poor were assisted by taxes collected and administered at the local level. As in England, workhouses for the poor and apprenticeship programs were established. Both the New World and the Old showed a marked differentiation in their treatment of what they identified as the "worthy" versus the "non-worthy" poor. The worthy poor were seen as those who found themselves indigent and dependent through no fault of their own. Counted in the group of the worthy poor were widows, the physically ill, and dependent children. The "unworthy poor" were those in difficult straits caused, ostensibly, by their own choices and actions rather than unfortunate circumstances. This group generally included alcoholics, prostitutes, and malingerers. Although no longer referred to by these terms, society continues to maintain somewhat similar attitudes in determining who deserves assistance.

One of the first efforts assisting people in deprived or at-risk circumstances was the utilization of the "friendly visitor." Frequently middle-class women from the community, the friendly visitors sought out those in need and met with them in their homes. They assessed needs and attempted to help alleviate problems and hardships through advice and advocacy in social systems. Material help could be given to those considered "deserving," but the emphasis was on teaching people to help themselves. The first friendly visitors were volunteers from the community, with little, if any, formal training. Under the auspices of the Charity Organization Societies, the volunteers were the forerunners of today's social workers.

In the early 1900s, Mary Richmond was a monumental force in shaping and defining the field of social work. Richmond elucidated the principles of social casework and advocated for the professional training of social workers. Her *Social Diagnosis* is one of the archetypes of social work literature. She was one of the first to articulate a theory of social system that looked at the impact of the various subsystems to which a person belonged. These systems included family, personal, ethnic, community, and charitable. Richmond developed many standard questions to be asked of the client concerning the various social systems relevant to his or her situation. This represented a shift in focus from approaching the person with preconceived notions and solutions to enlisting the input and assistance of the person in defining individual needs.

During the past 50 years, social work has undergone a metamorphosis from its early days of community outreach. In their book, *Unfaithful Angels: How Social Work Abandoned Its Mission,* Specht and Courtney decry what they feel is the abandonment of social issues and the poor by the social workers. The central theme of *Unfaithful Angels* is the movement by many social workers away from community work and concrete services into the areas of individual psychotherapy and private practice.

In the book *Home Health and Rehabilitation*, edited by Dr. Bella J. May, Barbara Nowell Jackson documents the strong role that physical therapy plays in home health care today. Physical therapy is the second most frequently employed discipline in the home, second only to skilled nursing. This is quite a statement considering that skilled nursing care is a prerequisite to Medicare reimbursement. In a 1990 survey by the North Carolina Home Health Care Association, most home care patients received visits by skilled nurses, followed by 32% of visits made by physical therapists, edging out visits made by home health aides at 28%.

Although difficult to document, it seems that physical therapy got its start in home care when VNAs began proliferating. Nursing agencies realized the need for and benefit to their patients of incorporating physical therapy into the care plans of their patients. In the post-Medicare/Medicaid years, physical therapy has achieved a staggering rate of growth in the area of home health care. Physical and occupational therapists play an invaluable role in the recovery of the patient as they work to assist patients in regaining their physical capabilities.

Although a number of health care professionals, such as nurses, physicians, and social workers, routinely went into the home in the early 19th century, Moore states that the existence of large extended families often made the need for homemaker services, as we know them today, unnecessary. Moore also states that, in the 1920s, homemakers were used to provide care for families when the mother was either ill or away.

As with most home care services, the advent of Medicare and Medicaid greatly expanded the use of home health aides and homemakers. Moore believes that the Title XX funds made available by the Social Security Amendment Act of 1974 greatly contributed to the proliferation of these services both in the public and the private sector. In the 1970s, the demand for these services and the availability of funding helped to create a market for the for-profit companies and national chains. In 1994, The National Association for Home Care reports that there were more than 48,000 physical therapists working in the home. Numerically, only RNs numbering more than 250,000 and home health aides at 170,000 represented greater numbers in home care.

Home Care Declines

Following the Golden Age of home care—with physicians whose practices centered on their office and home visits and with Henry Street nurses and social workers who advocated the community delivery of health care to clients—home care went into a decline. In what seemed a natural evolution, health care moved from the home to the more scientifically sophisticated arena of the hospital. Here physicians and nurses could more closely control hygienic conditions and more fully use the advances being made in medical science. In essence, medicine underwent an Industrial Revolution all its own. It can be argued that what was gained in sterile technique and an almost miraculous ability to cure was lost in personal involvement and intimacy. The nature of the system defined a new type of health caregiver. Given large caseloads, and much time spent in the hospitals, the physician's home visit was becoming a thing of the past.

After about 50 years of little growth or change, the initiation of Medicare gave an enormous shot in the arm to the field of home health. Begun in 1965, Medicare provided reimbursement for a variety of skilled nursing and other services provided they were restorative in nature. As opposed to other services that were reimbursed at a rate of 80%, home services were covered 100%. An indication of the impact of Medicare coverage is apparent in the proliferation of home health agencies, which increased from barely more than 1,000 in 1963 to 15,000 today. In 1994, there were more than 650,000 home care workers providing care to 7 million Americans. This care involved costs exceeding $23 billion.

The American hospice movement added an important dimension to an emerging new era in home health care. Although VNAs and certainly many families and caregivers have always given care to the terminally ill at home, the growth of the hospice movement over the last 20 years has illuminated and humanized our treatment of the dying. Somewhere along the line we developed a largely unspoken assumption that if you were sick enough to die, you should be in a hospital. As most proponents of hospice are quick to point out, hospice is not a place, as it was in England where it began and in other countries, but rather a philosophy of care and program offered by health care organizations.

When restorative care is no longer feasible, the aim of hospice is to provide palliative care to the terminally ill in a manner that enhances the quality of their lives. As far back as the 5th century, there was a large hospice in Turmanin in Syria. At about the same time, St. Bridget provided hospice-type care to the dying in Ireland. Hospice continued to evolve through the Middle Ages with the Knights of Templar providing care not only for the ill and dying, but also for travelers, orphans, and the poor. Perhaps the most famous, and the prototype for much of the hospice care today, is St. Christopher's in London, founded by Dr. Cicely Saunders. A major proponent of hospice since the late 1960s, Dr. Elizabeth Kubler-Ross made staggering contributions to the understanding of the terminally ill with her book, *On Death and Dying*.

In 1975, a group of professionals in Marin County, California, who were familiar with the work of Drs. Saunders and Kubler-Ross, offered their services free of charge to dying members of the community. This grassroots effort was the seedling for the growing hospice movement now becoming the treatment of choice for many terminally ill Americans.

Not only is hospice a humane and noninvasive means of care, it saves much in health care costs. In *America's Health Care Revolution: Who Lives? Who Dies? Who Pays?*, Joseph A. Califano Jr., former Secretary of Health, Education, and Welfare, writes that at the time he was secretary of HEW, 30% of the Medicare budget was spent on those in their last year of life. "Why not cover care at home or in hospice, where an individual with terminal illness can die in dignity, with much of the pain relieved, holding the hands of his loved ones, rather than hooked to tubes, and plastic, and metal machines?" Califano asks.

The issue of our treatment of the dying affects us on both economic and humanitarian levels. While many areas of the economy have remained somewhat stagnant, home health care continues to experience significant growth. Estimates of this rate of growth range from 11% or 12% to as high as 35% per year.

Toward a New Definition of Home

Is home care the same today as when Lillian Wald's nurses climbed tenement stairs in turn-of-the-century New York? In some basic, primal way, yes. In many superficial ways, no. A time journey would indeed be a spectacular one for Wald and her constituents, including the founder of Planned Parenthood, community health nurse Margaret Sanger. To see the sophisticated wound care, intravenous therapies, "miracle" drugs, and modern prosthetic devices, as well as the ever-strengthening mind/body connection and theories of holistic care in action, would be a dream come true. One can't help but think that the development closest to Wald's heart might be the simple continuation of basic quality home care, from the patient recovering from simple surgery to the hospice patient maintained at home through the extraordinary advances in palliative care.

One of the great challenges facing home care today is the changing definitions of home and family. For the Henry Street nurses, home and family were fairly traditional, often stable commodities. Family generally consisted of the nuclear composition of mother, father, children, and possibly some extended family members or a boarder. Overcrowding may have indicated that several families shared a residence. Contemporary family structure is more a kaleidoscope of changing forms. There are more single-parent families, step-families, childless marriages, gay cohabitation and marriages, and single people than ever before. What constitutes home itself is also changing. Home may be a riverfront mansion or a converted chicken coop. It may be a boarding home, assisted living facility, high-rise apartment, trailer home, nursing home, or half-way house.

The horizon of home health care today is one of limitless opportunity. The privilege of meeting with the patient in his own home gives professionals and other caregivers a unique window on our patient's world and helps us join him on a level impossible in strictly clinical settings. Being in the patient's home enables us to assess more clearly the resources and supports available to our patients on material and emotional levels. In some fundamental way, that may always elude the grasp of scientific research. To interact with people in their own homes is to create a bond for both the patient and caregiver. Add to all these benefits the very real possibility that home care can provide excellent health care, meet the desire of the patient to remain at home, and at the same time considerably reduce formerly extravagant health care costs.

Coverage and the Cost Factor

Over the past 30 years, health care in the United States has undergone a metamorphosis. As medicine has developed a "Star Wars"–like technology, and social consciousness pushed toward expanding medical coverage in both the public and private spheres, we are faced with a monster created of our own good intentions. As President Clinton endeavors to develop a health care plan, even partisans seem prepared to admit there are no easy solutions. At this point, the United States has considerably outdistanced other developed nations in the amount of gross national product (GNP) consumed by health care. Since 1960, the percentage of GNP spent on health care in America has risen from slightly more than 5% to more than 12%. Great Britain appears to be the nation that has succeeded to the greatest extent in keeping a cap on these expenditures, having increased only from 4% to 6% over the same time period.

As Califano has beautifully documented in *America's Health Care Revolution,* public and private sectors laid the foundation for health care costs that would spiral beyond anyone's dreams. The analysis of Chrysler's efforts to appease union demands with what were considered to be minor health care benefits escalated into financial liabilities that contributed to the undermining of Chrysler's solvency and an inability to compete with Japanese auto manufacturers. According to Califano, 1 of every 10 dollars of the price of Chrysler vehicles represented health care costs. In 1984, Chrysler was paying $460 million in health care costs for employees and retirees. These costs combined with the double-digit inflation, high interest, and stiff foreign competition of that period.

Interestingly, this dire situation that mirrored much of what was happening at the same time throughout the private sector had an innocuous beginning. In 1941, Chrysler agreed to concede to union demands for group health insurance. The insurance did not cover physicians' fees. Over the next several decades, Chrysler agreed during contract negotiations to various increases in basic coverage that included payment of physicians' fees and the Medicare deductible for retirees, and dental and vision benefits. The effect of this extensive coverage was an almost geometric progression of health care expenditures, and at the same time an insulation of consumers from the real nature of the cost of their own health care.

At the same time this total coverage was increasing, medical technology was also rapidly advancing. In 1985, myriad tests and procedures, unheard of in 1941, emerged. For example, magnetic resonance imaging (MRI), a single test that is excellent for diagnostic purposes, costs about $1,000. Although we have yet to find a cure for cancer, our treatment techniques have become increasingly sophisticated. We increase life expectancies with chemotherapy and radiation treatment and, in some instances, bone marrow transplants. The availability of these treatments, along with the insulation of the consumer from cost and the advancing age of the workforce, created a scenario for economic disaster. In addition, there was virtually no regulation of costs or length of treatment. Physicians simply submitted fees for services. Chrysler appears to have assumed that the funds they were allocating in health care concession would only increase incrementally as the cost of living did so. They failed to see that the very nature of the health care they were guaranteeing was changing. Because the unions viewed their relationship with Chrysler as adversarial, they attempted to get the maximum from the system. They failed to see that, in fact, their relationship with Chrysler was symbiotic. If Chrysler didn't do well, neither would they.

As divergent as Chrysler, the private sector, and the federal government seem, they were adversely affected by many of the same factors. In 1965, the federal programs of Medicare and Medicaid were initiated to provide basic health care services for the elderly and the poor and disabled. It is interesting to note that from 1977 to 1989 alone, government expenditures on health care increased 81% even after adjusting for inflation. Here, too, the Medicare and Medicaid systems were adversely affected by the same environmental and systemic factors that nearly brought about the demise of the Chrysler Corporation. What began as an effort by the Johnson Administration to continue the social policies of the New Deal was hit by a rapidly aging population and tremendous strides in technology.

Diagnostic Related Groups (DRGs)

In 1983, Congress created a system of payment for hospitals which identified 470 "diagnosis related groups," or DRGs, which provided guidelines for the treatment of various diseases and conditions. This effort at cost containment radically altered treatment and hospital stays and now figures prominently in hospital administration and care. Essentially, hospitals make money on patients discharged in less time than that allotted by the DRG, and lose money for those patients who stay longer. To ensure that these guidelines did not work to the detriment of the patient, Medicare was required to establish Peer Review Organizations that would monitor hospitals for quality control.

An interesting parallel between both the public and private sector is that for a long time, physicians and patients were insulated from the cost of services which were being provided. For instance, 30 years ago health care costs did not appear to be the tremendous cause of concern that they are today. At that time, although many people had insurance coverage for hospital costs, many were not covered for physicians' fees. This factor played an important role in cost containment by affecting care decisions made by the physician and the consumer.

Medicaid is in a similarly strange position with subscribers being entitled to unusual treatments such as vasectomy reversals and bone marrow transplants, but often unable to find a primary care physician. Here again, a vicious cycle occurs because Medicaid patients see no alternative but to go to emergency rooms for minor complaints such as sore throats at a highly inflated cost.

Unfortunately, a pervasive feeling exists that cost containment and quality care seem to be mutually exclusive. In "Healthcare Polarities:

Quality and Cost," it is noted that many people who perform services, as opposed to administrators, view cost containment as an enemy to high quality care.

In the private sector, the concept of managed care has gone a long way toward introducing a lean, almost management-by-objective philosophy into health care planning. Managed care is having tremendous impact upon the delivery of health care services and is creating a free market in this sector of the economy. And over the next few years, there will be a movement away from inpatient care to outpatient care centers. Many new movements toward outpatient centers appear to be the cost-reducing trend of the future.

According to Val J. Halamandaris, president of the National Association for Home Care (NAHC), based in Washington, D.C., home care is the wave of the future. In an article he wrote for *CARING Magazine*, a NAHC publication, Halamandaris outlined 20 reasons for home care:

1. *It is delivered at home.* There are such positive feelings that all of us associate with being home. Our home is our castle, our refuge from the storm. When we are not feeling well, most of us ask to go home. When we are feeling well, we enjoy the sanctity of our residences and the joy of being with our loved ones.
2. *Home care represents the best tradition in American health care.* Home health agencies were started as public agencies to seek out the poor and the needy who otherwise would go without care. No one was turned away. This is still true for most of America's home health agencies.
3. *Home care keeps families together.* There is no more important social value. It is particularly important in time of illness.
4. *Home care serves to keep the elderly in independence.* None of us wants to be totally dependent and helpless. With some assistance, seniors can continue to function as viable members of society.
5. *Home care prevents or postpones institutionalization.* None of us wants to be placed in a nursing home unless this is the only place where we can obtain the 24-hour care that we need.
6. *Home care promotes healing.* There is scientific evidence that patients heal more quickly at home.
7. *Home care is safer.* For all of its lifesaving potential, statistics show that a hospital is a dangerous place. The risk of infection, for example, is high. It is not uncommon for patients to develop new health problems as a result of being hospitalized. These risks are eliminated when care is given at home.

8. *Home care allows a maximum amount of freedom for the individual.* A hospital, of necessity, is a regimented, regulated environment. The same is true of a nursing home. Upon admission to either, an individual is required to surrender a significant portion of his rights in the name of the common good. Such sacrifices are not required at home.

9. *Home care is a personalized care.* Home care is tailored to the needs of each individual. It is delivered on a one-to-one basis.

10. *Home care, by definition, involves the individual and the family in the care that is delivered.* The patient and his family are taught to participate in their health care. They are taught how to get well and how to stay that way.

11. *Home care reduces stress.* Unlike most forms of health care, which can increase anxiety and stress, home care has the opposite effect.

12. *Home care is the most effective form of health care.* There is very high consumer satisfaction associated with care delivered in the home.

13. *Home care is the most efficient form of health care.* By bringing health services home, the patient does not generate room and board expenses. The patient and/or his family supply the food and tend to the individual's other needs. Technology has now developed to the point where almost any service that is available in a hospital can be offered at home.

14. *Home care is given by special people.* By and large, employees of home health agencies look at their work not as a job or profession but as a calling. Home care workers are highly trained and seem to share a certain reverence for life.

15. *Home care is the only way to reach some people.* Home health care has its roots in the early 1900s when some method was needed to provide care for the flood of immigrants who populated our major cities. These individuals usually did not speak English, had little money, and did not understand American medicine. The same conditions exist now to some extent because of the new wave of immigrants and the large number of homeless individuals who roam our streets.

16. *There is little fraud and abuse associated with home care.* Other parts of the health care delivery system have been riddled with fraud and charges of poor care. There have been few, if any, major scandals related to home care.

17. *Home care improves the quality of life.* Home care helps not only add years to life, but life to years. People receiving home care get along better. It is a proven fact.

18. *Home care is less expensive than other forms of care.* The evidence of this is overwhelming. Home care costs only one-tenth as much as

hospitalization and only one-fourth as much as nursing home placement to deal with comparable problems.

19. *Home care extends life.* The U.S. General Accounting Office has established beyond doubt that those people receiving home care lived longer and enjoyed living.

20. *Home care is the preferred form of care, even for individuals who are terminally ill.* There is growing public acceptance and demand for hospice care, which is home care for individuals who are terminally ill.

Little wonder that the public is demanding that (home care) be made more available. It is an idea whose time has come. *(Used with permission of NAHC.)*

As we go to press, Medicare and Medicaid are up for legislation that can significantly change both systems. Over the past several months, the proposed changes have flip-flopped back and forth as lawmakers respond to the input from various interest groups.

Summary

- Health Care began in the home.

- Each of the health professions has a history of care in the home:
  - Medicine: "The House Call"
  - Nursing: William Rathbone, District Nurses, Lillian Wald and the visiting nurse, Kelman, the Instructive Visiting Nurse.
  - Social Work: "The friendly visitor"
  - Physical Therapy: from Sister Kenny to the home
  - Dentistry
  - Nutritionists and Dietitians
  - Speech Therapy
  - Physical Therapy
  - Occupational Therapy
  - Respiratory Therapy

- Hospitals came into being with the Industrial Revolution and the use of the sterile field.

- Health care is moving aggressively toward outpatient care, with much of that care being performed in the home.

- In 1963, there were approximately 1,000 home care agencies; today, there are 15,000.

- Most health care professions offer little, if any, preparation for working in the home.

- Limitations on lengths of stay in hospitals have greatly increased the need for home care because patients are discharged while still in need of significant professional care.

- Home care represents a new frontier and offers unique opportunities in health care to contain costs while meeting a desire many patients have to stay at home.

- About 15,000 providers, including nurses, social workers, chaplains, physical and occupational therapists, and home health aides deliver home care services to more than 7 million individuals who have acute illnesses, long-term health conditions, permanent disability or terminal illness.

- As lifestyles change, there is a corresponding change in the definition of what constitutes "home." Home has been expanded to include nursing homes, boarding homes, shelters for the homeless, long-term care facilities and other places a person might call home.

Whose Home is it Anyway? Starting Where the Client Is

Home is the place where, when you have to go there,
They have to take you in.
Robert Frost

Half to forget the wandering and pain,
Half to remember days that have gone by,
And dream and dream that I am home again!
James Elroy Flecker

An Englishman's house is his castle.
from J. Ray's English Proverbs, 1670

Mrs. Ross, an 85-year-old widow, lives in a high-rise senior citizen apartment building. She is being seen by the visiting nurse for uncontrolled hypertension. Although very independent, she has become forgetful and left pots burning on the stove that set off fire alarms and create a hazard for other residents.

Mr. Grant is a 50-year-old merchant seaman who lives in a studio apartment in a former seaside hotel. He had surgery for bleeding ulcers and returned home still very weak. Before the operation, Mr. Grant had gone out for his meals. The health care team is concerned about his ability to recover without some assistance.

Ms. Walsh is a 40-year-old woman who lives in a single room occupancy (SRO) and has diabetes. She has had substance abuse problems for many years and frequently forgets to take her insulin. The emergency squad in the small town where she lives has taken her to the emergency room 59 times in the past year. The trips have incurred tremendous expense for the hospital and the town. In one instance, another resident died of cardiac arrest while the ambulance was transporting Ms. Walsh.

Mr. Harvey has been operated on for lung cancer and is being seen by the visiting nurse. He is taking many drugs, but he continues to smoke and drink heavily.

Mrs. Marks, 90, is a member of a prominent, wealthy family. She lives alone in a rambling old mansion in need of many repairs. Mrs. Marks has Alzheimer's disease and has fallen several times and been seriously hurt. The social worker contacted her son, who is politically active and owns several businesses in the community. Mr. Marks says that his mother has had a few falls that "could happen to anyone," and he really feels the health care agency should keep out of it.

Ms. Walker is a 33-year-old mother who has AIDS. Her daughters are 16 and 4, and her son is 12. Although she may live only six more months, she has only told the children that she has pneumonia. She has made no plans for their future.

Whose home? Whose life? Whose illness? And last, but possibly most important, who decides? All of the case scenarios above bring up questions we ask daily in home care. When we say a person's home is his castle, one can almost hear the braggadocio of Ralph Kramden in the old television series "The Honeymooners": "And I'm the king of the castle, Alice! The king!" Despite Ralph's comedic roaring, he tapped into an elemental truth. What he verbalized was that it didn't matter whether it was a cold-water flat or a penthouse on Park Avenue: A person's control in his or her own home is virtually limitless.

An interesting shift in this basic tenet of American life takes place, however, when the locus of control moves from the hospital to the patient's home. In the hospital, there is little equivocation about who is in control. The Patient's Bill of Rights enumerates important rights that are guaranteed to hospital patients, for example, the right to know what medication they are being given. But the patient does abdicate many things in exchange for the care a hospital provides. Some of the rights temporarily relinquished may seem insignificant, but for many people they are inextricably tied to a sense of autonomy and self-determination.

For openers, consider that the hospital staff decides when the patient will get up, when she will eat, when she will go for physical therapy, and when she may have visitors. Being compelled to awaken before dawn for preoperative assessment and preparation, or for a priest who marches in with Holy Communion, can make one's own home seem as pampering as Club Med.

While staying in the hospital requires compliance with the house rules, the rules are one's own at home. Given the logistics of providing medical care to a large number of people in one location, regimentation in the hospital or care facility is necessary. But the sacredness of a person's home affords a different philosophical approach for caregivers. It is sobering to realize that the law protects the integrity of the home even in relation to itself by prohibiting illegal searches and prosecuting criminal intruders.

The Client's Bill of Rights

1. Every patient's civil and religious liberties, including the right to make independent personal decisions and have knowledge of available choices, shall not be infringed, and the facility shall encourage and assist in the fullest possible exercise of these rights.
2. Every patient shall have the right to have private communications and consultations with his physician, attorney, and any other person.
3. Every patient shall have the right to present grievances on behalf of himself or herself or others to the facility's staff or administrator, to government officials, or to any other person without fear of reprisal, and to join with other patients or individuals within or outside of the facility to work for improvements in patient care.
4. Every patient shall have the right to manage his own financial affairs, or to have at least a quarterly accounting of any personal financial transactions undertaken in his behalf by the facility during any period of time the patient has delegated such responsibilities to the facility.
5. Every patient shall have the right to receive adequate and appropriate medical care, to be fully informed of his medical condition and proposed treatment unless medically contraindicated, and to refuse medication and treatment after being fully informed of and understanding the consequences of such actions.
6. Every patient shall have the right to privacy in treatment and in caring for personal needs, confidentiality in the treatment of personal and medical records, and security in storing personal possessions.
7. Every patient shall have the right to receive courteous, fair, and respectful care and treatment and a written statement of the services provided by the facility, including those required to be offered on an as-needed basis.

8. Every patient shall be free from mental and physical abuse and from physical and chemical restraints, except those restraints authorized in writing by a physician for a specified and limited period of time or as are necessitated by an emergency, in which case the restraint may only be applied by a qualified licensed nurse who shall set forth in writing the circumstances requiring the use of the restraint and in the case of use of a chemical restraint a physician shall be consulted within 24 hours.

9. Every patient has the right to a statement of the facility's regulations and an explanation of the patient's responsibility to obey all reasonable regulations of the facility and to respect the personal rights and private property of the other patients.

Excerpted from the New York Public Health Law 2803, McKinney, 1987.

Many facilities and home health agencies have a clients' or patients' bill of rights tailored to their services and policies. The Client's Bill of Rights mandates certain actions on the part of the health care agency to ensure the preservation of basic patients' rights in the home setting. By requiring that patients are made aware of and consent to the presence of staff members in their homes, that they be informed of any additional charges that will be incurred by placing equipment or services in the home, and also that they be given information regarding advanced directives, the Client's Bill of Rights safeguards the patient's rights both as a person and consumer. These rights provide a framework for the caregiver as well.

Never married, Mr. Miller, 75, was a history teacher and has been retired for 10 years. He lives in a cottage on a lake with many books and an aging beagle, Gustav, and a cockatoo named Darwin. Retirement has been wonderful. Mr. Miller traveled whenever he had opportunity, played golf and bridge, and read all the books he's wanted to read. When Mr. Miller was sent for a chest x-ray after a persistent cold, a spot on his lung was discovered. Diagnosed with cancer, he was treated at the local hospital with chemotherapy and sent home with a referral to the local VNA.

His first day home, he was visited by the nurse who was to develop a plan of care for him. He was to be seen by the nurse three times a week; the physical therapist was scheduled for a weekly visit, a social worker's visit was scheduled, and a home health aide was to come five times a week for two hours. Mr. Miller, who has lived a quiet, scholarly life, and Gustav, who is quite antisocial, are totally overwhelmed by this disruptive "parade."

Simple Considerations

As health care workers, first and foremost we are guests in our clients' homes. While we meet our patients in a time of crisis, we should do our best to help restore normalcy and assuage their stress. Some basic rules may work to establish mutual trust and consideration.

- Explain the roles of other team members and how they will assist the patient.
- As much as possible, respect the patient's wishes for scheduling appointments.
- If you're going to be late, call. If you have to cancel, give as much notice as possible.
- Make sure that the patient or caregiver knows how to get in touch with the agency.
- Work with patients' different needs and styles. Some patients may need more support and take more time, whereas others may just want the visit to end as quickly as possible.
- As much as possible, be accepting of other lifestyles and standards of living.

Establishing a Plan of Care

Establishing a patient's plan of care is truly a collaborative effort. The most sophisticated care plan will be little more than an academic exercise if the patient doesn't see its value. Jerry Carter has contributed tremendously to the field of social work and human service with his "Life of a Group," a dramatic presentation of the workings and evolution of the therapeutic group. He recounts a personal anecdote that shows how the goals of the caregiver and the patient can be light years apart.

A young, inexperienced social worker working with families in the Appalachian mountains, Carter arrived impeccably dressed in a new suit and overcoat to visit a family living in a squalid, two-room shack. The father was dying of lung cancer. Eager to help, Carter began to set forth some solutions for this family. But he encountered a problem: The solutions he proposed were not even close to the solutions the family wanted. Even their perception of the problem was worlds apart from his.

While Carter opted to develop a behavior modification program to help the father stop smoking, the father aggressively sought ways to get more cigarettes. The relationship between the social worker and the family continued like this until Carter, who was to become a superb clinician, realized you can lead a horse to water, but you'd better not try to stick his head in it.

Part of the beauty of Jerry Carter's story is that we can all see ourselves as helpers. We have the solutions. We know what to do. Now, if these patients would just listen to us, everything would be fine. We become victims of our zealous desire to help, and in so doing, forget the patient's world. As Carter admirably points out, a caregiver may be like the proverbial Boy Scout who is astonished when the elderly lady he's "escorted" across the street hits him with her umbrella.

How do we establish common ground? "Start where the client is" is one most frequently invoked axioms of social work and possibly the most valuable. You know your definition and solution to the problem. Now explore what the patient sees as the problem. What is he or she willing to do to bring about a solution? What is his concept of a solution? In home care, the referral to a patient is made because the physician or social worker believes it is necessary. Some questions that may help create an understanding of the patient's perception of the situation include:

- How do you think home care services can help you?
- Have you had home health services before?
- If so, were they helpful?
- What was most helpful? What was least helpful?

If you listen carefully, you may be surprised at what you learn. A caregiver may be astounded at how different a patient's goals might be from the professional caregiver's goals. Whatever you discover will bring you that much closer to being able to help your patients.

Case 1

Mrs. Jones, a hospice patient, with lung cancer and metastasis to the bone, has a prognosis of six months.
Patient goal: Mrs. Jones, an avid gardener all her life, would like to be able to transfer to a wheelchair so she can sit in her garden.
Caregiver goal: The hospice team would like to maintain Mrs. Jones so she is as comfortable as possible without aggressive treatment and promote her quality of life.

Case 2

Mrs. Wilson and her developmentally disabled son, Jim, live on a dilapidated old farm. Mrs. Wilson cared for Jim totally until she suffered a fall and broke her hip.

Patient goal: Mrs. Wilson, who is extremely independent, wishes to remain in her home.
Caregiver goal: The health care team sees the need for Mrs. Wilson to keep her hip immobilized. The team wishes to see care delivered in a safe, monitored environment.

Case 3

Mr. Watson, 69, suffers from severe emphysema. He lives alone and is being seen by the visiting nurse. He is no longer able to drive.
Patient goal: Mr. Watson would like the agency social worker to procure transportation to take him to the bar where he has had lunch and spent the afternoon drinking for the past four years.
Caregiver goal: The visiting nurse and social worker would like Mr. Watson to give up smoking and begin to cultivate healthier habits.

Agreement of Goals

Obviously, some of these goals are similar, while others are miles apart. The first step in the process of arriving at agreement is to establish a dialogue. After determining how the patient defines his or her own needs, what is important, what he values, and how close his "wish list" is to the realistic treatment goals, the caregiver needs to let the patient know what can be provided.

The treatment of each patient must be highly individualized. Patients present care needs varying from the simple and mundane to the multifaceted and seemingly insoluble. In a similar manner, patients' knowledge of home care may range from the sophisticated to nearly non-existent. Furthermore, what patients expect or want from home health services will vary as much. As the caregiver determines where the patients fall on this continuum, a baseline from which to develop a plan of care emerges.

The foundation of the plan of care is agreement between the health care provider and the client as to what needs to be done and how it will be accomplished. In *The Tao of Negotiation*, Edelson and Crain describe different strategies for eliciting clarity in communication. After you have a sense of how clients see the problem and what they would like to see happen, you need to do the following.

Clarify Your Role

Let the patient say what you can and cannot do for him. One way to think of this is to share with the client an informal job description. Example for a physical therapist: "I am going to work with you so you can transfer into the wheelchair." This strategy is helpful especially when someone wants you to mail letters, iron curtains, take out the dog, or lie to his boss. When you are engaged in this part of the process, remember that although the parameters of your job or responsibility are very clear to you, most patients have had little exposure to them.

In the world of home care, a patient may feel like a stranger in a strange land. Often the patient may not initially see how the physical therapist differs from the home health aide or the nurse. A patient may have even less of an idea of what the social worker can do for her. Here you essentially function in the role of educator, explaining to the patient your specific role and that of the home care agency. Keep your explanation concrete and simple. For the most part, patients may be overwhelmed and dealing with information overload. Whenever possible, operationalize roles. For example, a caregiver may say, "The home health aide will be here from 9 to 11 a.m. on Monday, Wednesday and Friday. He (or she) will give you your bath and do your laundry."

Assess the Role Significant Others Play in the Patient's Care

The patient's spouse, relatives, significant others, and community affiliations play an important part in the patient's recovery. As a caregiver, it is important to know how these significant others will participate in the care. It is also important to realize that frequently a significant other may fall outside the formally recognized and traditional roles. Consider, for instance, Mr. W., 48, who lives in a small boarding home. Mr. W. was a successful stock broker until he had a nervous breakdown following the death of his wife and two small children in a car accident. He never worked again. Although he had no biological family, he was loved in the boarding home for his gentle manner and willingness to help. For Mr. W., the boarding home residents constituted a family of choice. As he became progressively ill with lung cancer, the boarding home residents provided him with a variety of support, from supplying him with books to keeping him company, and the boarding home owner drove him for his chemotherapy and doctor's appointments.

At times, a patient may designate a significant other to receive information for him. For example, he may tell a significant other, "Please tell my son or daughter that." The patient may be relying upon the significant other because he feels stressed and overwhelmed, or it may be a role the significant other has long filled in his life. In either case, it is important to respect the patient's wishes.

It is also important to get a sense of how the patient's illness will affect his or her significant others. The patient's illness may have an impact on many areas of the person's life — the financial to the emotional to the social. An elderly person may be a caregiver for an elderly, incapacitated spouse. A young mother may be responsible for the care and well-being of several preschool-age children. The person who has no significant others is possibly the one who presents the greatest challenge to home care services.

Share with Patients Your Assessment of Their Needs and What You Envision as a Plan of Care

Here you give the patient your therapeutic evaluation, describe interventions, and give treatment goals. Despite the fact that this is your best professional assessment, let the patient know that recovery is a dynamic process with many rises and falls and that nothing is written in stone. In the case of Mrs. Jones, the patient who wishes to transfer to the wheelchair, the physical therapist can tell the patient what therapeutic interventions are necessary, how long treatment will take, and what circumstances will positively or negatively alter outcomes.

Elicit the Client's Input Regarding the Accuracy of the Assessment and Care Plan

If the patient basically concurs with your assessment and treatment plan, you have a starting point. If the patient sees his or her situation in a much different light, discuss the concerns. The patient's concerns may give you additional information that will change both your assessment and plan of care. In the event that a patient's goals seem extremely unrealistic, be honest. The patient needs to know what you feel you can and cannot accomplish. Unless you deal with these issues, they may surface later and undermine the patient's trust and your credibility. At this point, you need to explain why it is not a reasonable goal. You can then go on to what you believe you can accomplish. These actions, it is hoped, will bring you closer to agreement.

Check to See That Your Understanding of the Plan of Care and the Client's Understanding are the Same

There are a great many variables that can interfere with the patient's comprehension of the information you have given. To begin with, he or she is ill, stressed, possibly in an entirely new situation, and unfamiliar with many of the concepts you are trying to convey. To make sure a client understands thoroughly and agrees with the plan of care, restate it.

If you have any doubts as to why this is necessary, simply think back to a recent doctor's visit. Think of how many times you have come home and realized you are still unclear about a direction given or something that was said. Reiterating what you have discussed with a client reduces misunderstandings—a benefit for you and the patient. If you are in agreement, you have the skeleton of the care plan, and you have established the reason for being a welcome guest in your client's "castle."

Basic Ethical Considerations

What do we owe our patients? The most important ethical consideration is the primacy of the patient's care. The care and well-being of our clients is the focus of our work, and everything else from agency policy to personality conflicts becomes secondary. The field of medical ethics gives us several precepts for providing care:

1. *Autonomy and self-determination.* The concept of autonomy relates to the individual's ability to choose the best course of action for his care. To ensure autonomy and self-determination, the health care provider must see that the patient has the information necessary to make an informed decision. Once the person has the information needed, we must safeguard the right of the patient to make that decision. Finally, any information or knowledge of the patient is protected by confidentiality. A nurse who had worked with children for many years defines confidentiality as a "good secret." Information regarding a patient may not be conveyed to another without the consent and knowledge of the patient. Generally, a patient will be informed that confidentiality may be broken if there is danger present either to the client or another person.
2. *Beneficence/non-maleficence.* These are concepts that lie at the heart of all good health care. They refer to the basic obligation to do no harm, prevent harm and promote the well-being of our clients.

3. *Justice and equity*. These concepts relate to the obligation to promote an adequate level of care for all patients and to see that all patients are treated equitably.
4. *The integrity of the health care professional*. As professionals, we must adhere to a high level of practice as mandated by our respective disciplines. In conjunction with this, if we have personal or religious conflicts that will prevent us from performing certain types of care, we need to make these known to the appropriate people.

Abusive or Dangerous Situations

Caregivers may all too frequently encounter situations that are abusive or dangerous. The 84-year-old widow who leaves pots burning on the stove, the man with lung cancer who continues to smoke and drink, the wealthy dowager who stumbles around the mansion unattended are all situations that are difficult to deal with morally, ethically, and professionally. These situations bring up issues of autonomy, self-determination, and issues of safety for the individual and others. Some of the dangerous and abusive situations that may be encountered by the caregiver include financial exploitation, physical abuse or battery, and self-neglect (see Chapter 3 for additional information).

Financial exploitation refers to a person who is being taken advantage of for another's personal gain. A possible scenario is the elderly person who is cultivated for his pension or social security checks and given little in the way of care. Physical abuse, although most often associated with the problems of women, can target anyone as a potential victim. Until recently, people did not ordinarily realize that husbands or boyfriends could also be victims of abuse.

Victims of physical abuse frequently attempt to keep the abuse a secret out of shame or a fear of retaliation. A health care worker has an obligation to provide for the total well-being of his or her patients. There are a variety of organizations that can help those who are abused. Most communities have shelters for battered women and protective services for the elderly.

Caregivers cannot afford to have "tunnel vision." They must take into account a client's total life situation to give a client individualized and effective care. When you are the only person who stands between a person being abused and a resource for help, you must assess your own resources and find ways to set them in motion on behalf of your client. In short, caregivers must be brave but not foolhardy. Compassion is paramount.

Summary

- Initial referrals are generally made by a hospital discharge planner and must be ordered by a physician. Referrals may come from a variety of other sources such as word of mouth, health fairs, school personnel, or community organizations or case finding.

- The registered nurse visits the home and makes an initial assessment of patient needs. This visit includes gathering baseline data and information and performing a nursing evaluation.

- The nurse also uses the initial visit to begin to establish a therapeutic relationship. The most important outcome of the initial visit is contracting with the patient regarding services to be provided in the home.

- In addition to information-gathering, the initial visit is essentially educational. The nurse:
  1. assesses patient needs
  2. actively involves the patient in this process
  3. establishes a preliminary plan of care
  4. shares this with the patient and explains what will be done, by whom and when
  5. reaches agreement with the patient regarding professional, patient and caregiver responsibilities

- While many patients are familiar with some hospital procedures and routines, relatively few have experienced a home-care situation. The information may be difficult to absorb all at once.

- Pending approval by the physician, the nurse is the case manager and decides long- and short-term treatment goals, what services will be provided and for what length of time. This plan of care will be kept both in the home and the health care agency.

- The nurse designates appropriate services and makes referrals to these disciplines. While each agency has its own policies and methods, usually the nurse informs others of various disciplines of the reason for referring and expected outcomes of this referral.

- Throughout the course of treatment, the nurse and other team members confer to evaluate treatment outcomes.

Beyond the Melting Pot: Diversity and the Caregiver

If we cannot end now our differences, at least we can help make the world safe for diversity.
John F. Kennedy, 1963 address at American University, Washington, D.C.

There were never in the world two opinions alike, any more than two hairs or two grains. Their most universal quality is diversity.
Montaigne, *Essays*

If God wanted everyone to be alike, we'd all be wearing braces.
Winston Groom, *Forrest Gump*

A young physical therapist anxiously looks at her watch. It is early in the morning as she drives in a dense fog along an unmarked back road, an anomaly in an otherwise suburban area. She counts the houses — former chicken or sheep farms — before arriving at a somewhat rickety house that matches the description of the one in which her client lives. At the door, she is greeted by an unsmiling woman in her late 50s, who leads her into the bedroom of her husband. When the man sees the physical therapist's black hair and dark skin, he immediately tells his wife he does not want the young woman's services and to get him another therapist. By now, the therapist recognizes the need for composure. Surprised and offended, she excuses herself politely.

A nurse's aide was sent by the registry to the home of an Asian woman who has had several strokes and may have organic brain syndrome. The woman, who spoke broken English, was unreasonable, demanding that the nurse's aide cook with unfamiliar Asian ingredients and never sit down. Whenever the nurse's aide tried to help her patient, the woman became combative. After one shift, the aide felt unable to continue the assignment. She also told the registry she was unwilling to care for any other Asian patient.

When poet Emma Lazarus wrote, "Give me your tired, your poor, your huddled masses yearning to breathe free," she spoke to the heart of public health and public health nursing. The focus of home health care has always been to bring quality health care to those in need, regardless of their ability to pay. From its inception in the Henry Street Settlement to the large VNAs of today, home health care has not wavered from this mission.

In applying for my first job in home care, the supervisor who interviewed me told me that 70% of the patients cared for by the agency were older than 70, a significant number lived in high crime areas, many were poor, a sizable number had problems with substance abuse, many were multiply handicapped, and the patient population represented just about every ethnic and racial group. She said if any of these variables was a problem, this was not the job for me. It posed an illuminating question. While I had never considered myself to be a prejudiced person, suddenly the number of prejudices human beings can harbor seemed vast. It occurred to me that the issue of prejudice was not a question of either/or, but very much one of degree. We can have very strong feelings about people because of their age, sex, race, whether they keep plastic ducks on their lawn, live in public housing, or have a bumpersticker that says, "Honk if you love Jesus." Whatever our feelings about a person's lifestyle, personality, political or religious affiliations, we have a sacred trust and a professional obligation to provide them with the highest level of care of which we are capable. For most of us, the process of professional growth continues throughout our careers.

— M.L.F.

It may seem audacious to approach an issue as volatile as diversity in one chapter. But its purpose is to touch — or at least to provide a thought-provoking springboard for further communication and sensitivity — on issues that affect professional and personal development and that continuously evolve over the course of a lifetime. Naturally, we do not intend to present stereotypes. Rather, we wish to encourage the celebration of individuality, that variable that is unknowable until one makes an effort to get to know it.

Mixed marriages all over the world also play a part in the "melting pot," fusing physical and personality traits. Stereotypes diminish constantly as people come together to create unique children. To invest in the image of the "somber, gruff northern German" and the "friendly, smiling Irish" triggers calamity for the caregiver (and probably anyone else), for certainly there are jovial northern Germans and somber, gruff

Irish. Immigration is an ongoing process, and American caregivers are daily introduced to previously unfamiliar ethnic groups and cultures. The key points to remember are:

1. Be open, observant, and sensitive.
2. Be aware that you seem different, too.
3. Be aware that some people may expect others to be biased against them.
4. Be an advocate for one who may not be familiar with the American health care system.
5. Be willing to spend more time with clients of other ethnic groups to establish trust and meet needs.
6. Anticipate differences on matters of illness, seeking help, death and dying, sexuality, spirituality, dress and grooming, food and eating habits, sense of personal space, time awareness, nonverbal communication, and relationships.
7. Give yourself credit for doing your best to be flexible.
8. Acknowledge the differences between your life experience and that of your client. Eliminate labels, misconceptions, and stereotypes.
9. Always celebrate the individual.
10. Kindness is universal.

Home care has always been dedicated to providing care to all people regardless of race, religion, sex, national origin, or ability to pay. If it is not considered so already, it should be an inalienable right. The issues of diversity that faced the Henry Street nurses and early social workers and that face contemporary home health workers are different in name and circumstance only: the underlying principle remains the same.

In the early 1900s, those in need of care may have been young immigrant families or individuals with tuberculosis. Today we may be caring for the terminally ill or the frail elderly. While technology has taken giant steps, the mission of health care also remains the same — to restore, rehabilitate, and maintain optimal well-being.

For many years, Americans subscribed to a "melting pot" theory of their culture. Their perspective presented a society in which ethnic groups became assimilated into the larger society, and thus blended to form a homogeneous culture. Daniel Patrick Moynihan and Nathan Glaser contributed significantly to the understanding of ethnicity in America with their book, *Beyond the Melting Pot*. They advanced the theory that ethnic groups did not simply adopt or assimilate into the American culture, but that they adapted to the new culture as they retained many aspects of their specific culture. In *Beyond the Melting Pot*, the authors examine the immigration of the Irish, Germans, Jews, blacks, and Puerto Ricans to New York City, and they identified distinct cultural patterns and experiences.

Many sociologists have moved away from the "melting pot " theory of ethnicity to a belief that many ethnic groups retain aspects of their culture of origin for many generations. In the *Cultural Evolution of American Indian Families,* John Red Horse proposes a variety of family types that exist within the larger culture. Red Horse points out that these patterns are not linear and do not follow a set order, but rather indicate a system that is appropriate for that particular family and its circumstances. The patterns described by Red Horse would seem to be universal and are helpful in understanding the adaptive behaviors and differences within other ethnic and cultural groups and, more importantly, in understanding why patients, apart from individual differences, within the same ethnic group may exhibit behaviors that range from being highly cohesive with those of their ethnic group to mildly cohesive or even rejecting.

Traditional Families

These families identify to a high degree with cultural norms espoused by the ethnic or cultural group. Generally, family members are most comfortable with their native language. Extended kin relationships are often important in these families.

Neotraditional Families

Native language is generally preferred, however, some members may begin to acquire second-language proficiency. There may also be some adoption of mainstream cultural practices. For the most part, identification with the native group is strong, and there is a preference for affiliations with members of this group.

Transitional Families

Members use native language with family and close friends. Typically, members are proficient in use of English and use it extensively outside of the home and community environment. Members may travel to their country of origin to maintain contact with the culture from which they are becoming increasingly distant.

Bicultural Families

Members are increasingly involved in activities and organizations outside their native culture. English is generally used, but members will still have extensive involvements with people of their native culture. Children are not likely to be fluent in the native language. There may also be a decline in extended family networks.

Acculturated Families

In these families, there is usually little knowledge of native language and cultural practices. Here, members may often identify more strongly with the mainstream culture than with their ethnic culture. Family members may either convert to another religion or cease to practice the former. At times, there may be a tendency to see involvement in the native culture as a hindrance to success in the mainstream culture.

Panrenaissance Families

Behaviors of these family members may seem to constitute a reaction against a loss of cultural identification and involvement. Frequently, members have been brought up with little exposure to ethnic practices and seek ways to become more knowledgeable and participate in cultural activities. Members will often seek opportunities to learn the native language, spend time in the country and wish to be identified as a member of this culture. Some examples of this type of behavior include people pursuing studies in the Holocaust or joining a church specifically associated with an ethnic group.

As is well noted in ethnic literature, members of the same family may exhibit very different adaptive behaviors. For instance, one member of the family, typically a parent, may represent the traditional orientation exemplified by strict adherence to cultural norms, whereas another family member, frequently a child, may acquire the acculturated mode of behavior, characterized by efforts to identify and conform with the mainstream culture. These differences in adaptive behaviors are likely to set the stage for the inter-generational conflict between the young person's attempt to adopt the new culture and the parents' needs to preserve and honor their own culture. In working with patients of any culture, it is helpful to recognize the various ways in which people relate to their culture and also to be aware that people may shift their behavior patterns during different periods in their lives.

In this book, we offer a glimpse of some of the groups Moynihan and Glaser targeted as examples of what might be helpful information to the caregiver in an increasingly diverse society. Included also are special populations, such as the elderly, children, the mentally ill, the disabled, individuals with AIDS, the homeless, and gays and lesbians.

Gay and Lesbian Individuals

"Why do they hate us? Why do they fear us? Why do they want us invisible?" This quote is taken from Paul Monette's autobiography, *Becoming a Man: Half a Life Story*, which describes Monette's own struggle growing up gay in America. Until 1973, the American Psychiatric Association listed homosexuality as a psychiatric disorder. Although many organizations denounce discrimination based on sexual preference, in reality, the position of gay people is often precarious; for example, the continuing issue of gays in the military and the exclusion of gays from the annual New York St. Patrick's Day Parade. In health care, there is no equivocation.

Although approximately 10% of the population is gay, society is still homophobic. Bianca Cody Murphy notes in "In Educating Mental Health Professionals about Gay and Lesbian Issues," and article in the *Journal of Homosexuality*, "The majority of people in the United States see gay men and lesbian women as sick, immoral, criminal, or all three. Herek (1989)." In recent surveys, as many as 92% of lesbians and gay men report that they have been the targets of anti-gay verbal abuse or threats, and as many as 24% report physical attacks because of their sexual orientation.

In her article, Murphy calls for improvement of the education of health care professionals in gay issues and also in community resources for gay and lesbian clients. Another concern that looms large for the gay community is the lack of recognition of the gay person's significant other in health care issues and decisions because of the seemingly informal nature of the relationship. Often a person who has functioned as a spouse without the benefit of a legal document or a societally acknowledged bond will be extricated from or ignored in the event of a medical crisis.

The gay community has been extremely hard hit by the AIDS epidemic. In *And The Band Played On*, Randy Shilts chronicles the emergence of AIDS in this country. Here, the first question asked will be, "How did they get AIDS?" Society appears to feel very differently about people with AIDS based on the manner in which they contracted it. The least culpable tend to be those who contracted it through blood transfusions, probably followed by heterosexuals to whom it was transmitted by a marriage partner. For those who contract the disease either through intravenous drug use or homosexual contact, there is likely to be less compassion. The disease, however, shows no impartiality in the devastation it heaps upon the afflicted. The 53-year-old housewife who contracts AIDS from a blood transfusion related to a hysterectomy faces the same terrible road as the 26-year-old homeless drug user.

Multiple Losses and Guardianship Issues

We are dealing with a primarily young population who will be coping with losses that are atypical for their part of the life cycle. For example, we may have a 30-year-old male who suffers the loss of his job, his income, and his friends. In addition, there is the devastating societal stigma attached to AIDS. The stigma may lead to social isolation, secrecy, and refusal to reveal or attempts to identify the disease as something else, which is not uncommon for parents who try to protect their children. As one can easily imagine, this subterfuge carries with it an entire series of its own problems, including a sense of isolation and fear of being discovered.

AIDS

The AIDS epidemic has been health care's equivalent of the sinking of the Titanic: it wasn't supposed to happen. Just as the Titanic, regarded as a wonder of engineering, was thought unsinkable, the "Plague of the '80s" that systematically destroyed the immune systems of young, healthy people seemed to many more like science fiction than reality. As we are well into the second decade of this medical nightmare, a cure remains elusive. The good news is that many persons with AIDS are remaining healthier longer.

Issues for Caregivers of Patients with HIV/AIDS

CONTAGION

The viewpoint of the medical community regarding the transmission of the AIDS virus is extremely clear: The AIDS virus is not transmitted through casual contact, eg, shaking hands, using the same glass, or being in the same room. For medical personnel who will be involved in procedures that are more invasive in nature, the implementation of universal precautions will prevent contagion. Although these guidelines deal effectively with the concrete issues involved, they do not address the culture of fear that has grown around the emergence of this devastating disease. For many people growing up in the "Golden Age of Medical Technology," the appearance of AIDS was a health care nightmare that, it was hoped, would be short-lived. Those who believed in the invincibility of science awaited a cure from the arsenal of super-drugs. It is yet to come. This created a crisis in faith for those who believed that there is little that modern day science is not able to conquer.

The Centers for Disease Control and Prevention reports that AIDS is the fifth leading cause of death for women of child-bearing years. To further complicate the issue, 4,570 of the 213,641 reported AIDS cases from March 1990 to February 1992 were contracted via blood transfusion. (U.S. Department of Health and Human Services, Centers for Disease Control and Prevention, 1992.) The credibility of the health care community, which had believed in the safety of the blood supply, was compromised. The gap in credibility led many in the health care professions and the public to speculate that if they had erred with regard to the blood supply, they might also be wrong in determining how AIDS could be transmitted.

Perhaps few situations illustrate the tremendous fear incited by AIDS better than the case of Ryan White, and the attempt of Dr. Elizabeth Kubler-Ross to establish a hospice for babies with AIDS on her farm in Virginia. Ryan White, a young boy from Kokomo, Indiana, who contracted the AIDS virus following a transfusion for hemophilia, fought to remain in school following a school board decision to ban him from attending. Ryan White's courage and engaging personality made him an excellent representative for the struggle of people with AIDS. He died in 1990, but his legacy lives on in the federal grant program named for him that continues to provide assistance to people with AIDS. Because of severe community opposition similar to that which Ryan White encountered, Dr. Kubler-Ross eventually abandoned plans for the hospice.

It would be simplistic to assume that the people in these communities did not know the medical position on how AIDS is transmitted. It is more probable that many were aware of this position, but did not accept it. Or at the very least, they believed the risk involved was too great to accept the position entirely. Some of the fears expressed by health care workers include: What if they're wrong about how the AIDS virus is transmitted? Are we putting our family and loved ones at risk by working with people who are infected? What if a person is coughing profusely? Aren't health care workers simply at far greater risk because of the nature of their work?

WAYS OF DEALING WITH THESE FEARS

1. AIDS is a devastating disease. Realize that it is normal to be afraid.

2. Discuss your fears with colleagues and other support groups. You will realize that you are not alone.
3. As we move into the second decade of treating AIDS, the medical position regarding the transmission of AIDS is continually being proven accurate. We have not had occurrences of the virus from casual contact or when universal precautions are observed.
4. As with any infectious disease, be aware of the necessary precautions and observe them.

DEALING WITH THE PHYSICAL DEBILITATION OF AIDS

With the possible exception of cancer, few diseases can compare with AIDS in the physical devastation suffered by infected individuals. Because of the suppressed immune system, as the disease progresses a large number of opportunistic infections can occur: severe diarrhea, mouth sores, oral infections, Kaposi's sarcoma, and severe weight loss or wasting. The physical deterioration can be so extreme that it reminds one of Nazi concentration camp survivors. Seeing a patient with these symptoms can arouse a wide variety of emotions in the caregiver, including shock, pity, fear, and helplessness, a fear that our reactions will render us less able to help our patients. Whether we meet a patient already in a state of physical deterioration, or a patient who is in reasonably good health and who then begins to deteriorate, may mean the difference between facing an initial shock as opposed to the pain involved in watching someone physically decline.

COPING STRATEGIES

1. Get to know your patient. When you go beyond the superficial, ie, age, income, etc., and start to find out what is important to your patient — likes and dislikes, values, and personality — the physical aspects will take on less importance and become less difficult to deal with.
2. Cherish your ability to "feel bad." The ability to empathize is essential to caregiving.
3. Seek support from colleagues. Recognize that friends and family who are not involved in health care may not understand. Their responses may range from putting you on a pedestal, ie, "I don't know how you can do what you do," to "Why would you want to do something so depressing?"
4. Advocate for your patient. Whatever resources are available, whether medical, social or familial, help your patient acquire them.

One of the most heart-rending issues of the AIDS crisis is the increasing numbers of children who are being orphaned. These and others who may even be HIV-positive from birth may spend months in the hospital waiting for some resolution. One study advocates the implementation of an early intervention program for patients with HIV. This model includes a comprehensive assessment and case management component directed at addressing the varied needs that result from the disease. Areas that will be evaluated include HIV/AIDS-related education issues, coping abilities and support networks, financial needs, and long-term planning needs. The Ryan White Comprehensive AIDS Resources Emergency Act of 1990 provided millions for AIDS-related programs.

Through use of these federal funds, many states have specialized programs for persons with HIV/AIDS that provide numerous services. Frequently, the programs are administrated by local home health agencies or VNAs and offer medical, transportation, counseling, and homemaker services. The fastest growing group of persons with AIDS in the United States is women, and there has been an alarming increase in female adolescents with AIDS.

Discover Exactly Who Your Client Is

We have yet to arrive at the kind of world Dr. Martin Luther King, Jr. spoke of when he said, "I dream of a world in which people will be judged not by the color of their skin but by the content of their character." We may extend Dr. King's dream to include a world in which people are not judged by their sex, religious affiliation, ethnicity, or age. American society has been gifted with a unique mix of every race, ethnic, and religious group, and infinite types of lifestyles and political affiliations. The differences can be a source of joy and interest or the basis for prejudice and exclusion.

In the forthcoming decade, health care may find itself in a David-and-Goliath situation, with a monumental challenge in the area of fair distribution of health care resources. Skyrocketing costs pushed us further along the path to the rationing of health care resources and into a nation that must resolve its most difficult moral dilemmas in some acceptable way; for example, how do we decide how old a patient must be before it is no longer cost-effective to treat with chemotherapy? Who will be entitled to low-cost or free services of clinics and home health agencies? Who, in fact, comprise the disadvantaged, the disenfranchised, and vulnerable populations? The caregiver must realize that *any* person can be among those who are at risk of ill-health and ill-being. Let us begin to understand who we, the caregivers, are through the positive experience of discovering who our clients are.

Special Considerations for Health Care

ISSUES OF TRUST

In a historical context of broken agreements, issues of trust between American Indians and whites may well arise in health care situations. Attneave makes several suggestions to foster positive relationships. The most important of the suggestions is that the caregiver be him- or herself. Sincerity is probably the best tool to open the lines of communication. Developing an understanding of cultural practices is essential. Patients can be our greatest teachers. Other sources of information are cultural organizations and libraries.

ROLE OF THE TRADITIONAL HEALER

The healer, whether referred to as medicine person, shaman, or spiritual leader, has a pervasive function in American Indian culture. The activities are not limited to discrete medical roles but encompass also the spiritual and psychological aspects of one's being. Attneave notes cases in which traditional healing methods, such as use of a method similar to the "sweat lodge," were successful in the treatment of a case of alcoholism that did not respond to more conventional treatment. She records another history of prolonged grief that was resolved through the use of a ritual performed by a tribal healer. As health care providers, it is important to ascertain how the patient views these alternative methods and not assume what their views are.

John Red Horse reports the case of a young woman who lived for many years in a metropolitan area while she pursued her undergraduate and graduate degrees. During the seven years she lived there, she never went to a medical doctor, but rather returned home more than 60 times for ritual ceremonies for health-related issues.

In Paddy Chayefsky's play (and later the movie) "The Hospital," George C. Scott plays a physician who comes upon the bizarre sight and sounds of a Native American healer dancing and chanting around the hospital bed of an old man in a coma. Although the playwright pointed this out as an anomaly in the American hospital scene, such ritual healings, ethnic or general, may be destined to become as routine as a nurse bathing a patient.

CULTURAL AND TRIBAL DIFFERENCES

In establishing rapport with our patients, it is necessary to not only become aware of cultural practices, but also to become knowledgeable regarding their significance within a cultural context. For instance, the act of giving a gift to the health care provider is more meaningful in the American Indian culture than in other cultures.

Considerations for Practice

Because of the universal tendency to prefer the social system of family, friends and co-workers to outside organizations, it is beneficial for health care providers to work with the patient to use these networks as much as possible. Since there is often a reluctance to ask for help, it is especially important to try to elicit patient needs.

In conclusion, health care team members may incorporate into their practice Kluckhohn and Kroeber's excellent summary of the aspects of culture, which appear in Beare and Myers' book:

1. Culture is shared or learned, not biologically inherited. It is acquired after birth through experience.
2. Culture is inculcated or transmitted by passing the shared patterns of values, beliefs, customs, and behavior from one generation to the next (known as social enculturation).
3. Culture is social and relates to the interaction of individuals and groups.
4. Culture is ideational. Norms are traditionally acceptable ways that an individual should act in a given circumstance, although an individual may choose to behave otherwise. Actual behavior and expected behavior may differ and still be tolerated by one's cultural group.
5. Culture is gratifying. Members of a group find adherence to norms to be a satisfying experience. If members are not content with such standards, they will not perpetuate them.
6. Culture is adaptive. To survive, people must change to meet the changing demands of the environment. Also, a culture changes to adapt to its social and geographic surroundings, although changes are slow. This process is called acculturation. Immigrants coming to America are most often acculturated into this culture by the third generation.
7. Culture is integrative. All cultures have certain things in common related to the functions that all humans share in ordering their lives. Some of these universal aspects are religion, economics, communication patterns, values, beliefs, and customs. Each of these

elements can be assessed only in relation to each other. The overall nature of the culture is connected by the inter-relationship of each of these elements with one another.

The Disabled

The American with Disabilities Act of 1990 defines the disabled as individuals with physical or mental impairments that affect major life activities, those with a record of such conditions, or those who are perceived as having such disabilities. Included in this definition are the visually impaired, the wheelchair-bound, and those whose disabilities are not visibly identifiable, such as persons with psychiatric illness, AIDS, or a history of substance abuse.

The Americans with Disabilities Act is the most recent and comprehensive piece of legislation dealing with the rights of the disabled. The ADA prohibits discrimination in employment, public accommodation, public services, telecommunications, and transportation on the basis of disability by employers, businesses, and service providers in the public or private sectors. Furthermore, the Americans with Disabilities Act provides for the physical accommodation in public places, eg, ramps, for people with disabilities. The ADA superseded the previous law, which dealt only with buildings constructed with federal funds. The ADA has made compulsory many changes in buildings ranging from the small and privately owned buildings to the large public ones. The ADA lists the specific accommodations to be made for the hearing-, vision-, and physically impaired.

The Elderly

America is a youth-oriented society. Although Americans have been unfairly accused of "dumping" their elderly into nursing homes (the majority of the elderly are maintained at home, most frequently with the aid of a relative), we are not like many Asian, Pacific Island, and other societies that revere the elderly. Americans tend to resist the changes characteristic of advancing years, and our fear is seen in cultural oddities such as the "Over the Hill" party for a person turning 40. Deprived of the cultural supports present in other countries, the older years may be stressful. As Betty Friedan eloquently states in *The Fountain of Aging*: "It justifies the desperation to pass as young, to ward off the terror of aging. But as long as we acquiesce in that dread, as long as age itself is defined as sickness, doctors may not diagnose or even treat ailments in people over sixty-five that can be cured. And social workers, psycho-therapists, employers, and policy-makers will not deal with our real

41

needs and our real abilities for intimacy, work, involvement, respect, and self-respect, which may or may not be the same as the needs and abilities of the young, but nevertheless are vital to our lives."

In home care, approximately 70% of our clients will be older than 65, and this estimate may be conservative. As a group, the elderly possess unique strengths and have had unique life experiences. Many have lived through two World Wars, the Depression, and more technological changes than have occurred during the past 500 years. Most have completed many of the developmental tasks that society demands of its members; they have worked, married, maintained households, raised children, paid taxes, and contributed to community life.

Simply as a function of their developmental stage of life, older persons suffer a variety of losses, including the loss of job; change of social role; death of spouse, siblings, children, and long-time friends; a decrease in strength, agility, and sexual prowess; health problems; threats to economic stability; relocation from home; loss of personal freedom; a slowing of mental ability; alteration in self-image; and loss of acuteness of senses. Increasingly, many grandparents are functioning as, or taking over the role of, parent for their grandchildren. The litany of losses and possible difficulties is sobering.

The "Gray Ghetto"

Among the special problems of the elderly, and one of the frequently encountered scenarios in working with them, is the emergence of the "gray ghetto." Over time, a community originally composed of families and children may become radically changed when people die, move in with adult children in other areas, move to adult communities or nursing homes, or relocate to milder climates. Isolated and quite frequently fearful members of the community are the elderly who are left behind.

At the same time, the neighborhood may sustain an economic shift and may also fall prey to more socioeconomic problems and a higher crime rate, truly the places where the elderly may become prisoners in their own homes. They are often afraid to answer the door or the phone or go out after dark.

Elder Abuse

The National Aging Resource Center on Elder Abuse has identified seven categories of elder abuse, which include the following.

1. Physical abuse: nonaccidental use of physical force that results in bodily injury, pain, or impairment.

2. Sexual abuse: nonconsensual sexual contact of any kind with an older person.
3. Emotional or psychological abuse: willful infliction of mental or emotional anguish by threat, humiliation, or other verbal or nonverbal abusive conduct.
4. Neglect: willful or nonwillful failure by the caregiver to fulfill his or her caregiver obligation or duty.
5. Financial or material exploitation: unauthorized use of property, funds, or any resources of an older person.
6. Self-abuse and neglect: abusive or neglectful conduct of an older person directed at himself or herself that threatens his or her safety or health.
7. All other types: all other types of domestic elder abuse that do not belong to the first six categories.

The most prevalent type of documented abuse is self-neglect. The Older Americans Act (Part G, Title III) considerably widened the accepted definition of neglect by including "failure to provide for oneself." It should be well noted that in most states, health care workers are considered mandated reporters and are legally bound to report cases of suspected neglect. There are a few states that permit this reporting on a voluntary basis. Health care workers should become knowledgeable regarding the laws in their states.

The Elderly and Prescription Drugs

Because of the increase in physical ailments and conditions, the elderly are likely to be the segment of society that receives the most prescribed drugs. The high rate of prescription places the elderly at risk for a variety of complications ranging from possible drug interactions to, in some instances, addiction. Another danger that ensues from the high incidence of treatable conditions combined with the high cost of medication is prescription sharing.

The Homeless

Although we tend to think of homelessness as a social plague of the 1980s, we have seen variations of homelessness at different times in American history. During the Great Depression, many people who had lost their homes and their livelihoods lived like hobos on the outskirts of cities and towns. The dust bowl of 1936 — hundreds of thousands of acres of American farmland literally turned to dust as a result of prolonged droughts and dust storms — forced thousands of farmers and their families to search elsewhere for work and some type of opportunity. As economic conditions changed, many of these people were able to shake off the world of the homeless that had been theirs. In addition to an environmental type of crisis that induced homelessness, there was the more institutionalized homelessness of the Bowery. In the subcultures of society, people who "dropped out" of the mainstream found an "underground" culture. In the 1970s there was a dramatic rise in the rate of homelessness. Experts attributed this change to societal and political causes.

Clinics, governmental agencies, and home health agencies including VNAs tend to the multiple health-related and social needs of the homeless as much as possible. Many a home health caregiver travels each day to a single-room occupancy, a motel designated for the homeless, women's shelters and temporary residency programs, soup kitchens, drop-in sites, and other locations to provide care for individuals and families who find themselves adrift as a result of disenfranchisement, substance abuse, mental illness, and other problems.

The Mentally Ill

Most recently, the mentally ill are being moved out of the institution and into the community. Historically, the treatment of the mentally ill has determined the prevailing philosophies of care. Since the 1800s, the types of care afforded the mentally ill have changed drastically several times. Even the institution of Bedlam, England's Bethlehem Hospital that today is equated with a number of abuses including the use of physical restraints, bleeding, and the charging of admission to the public to view patients, represented an improvement over even more inhumane methods. As Ann Braden Johnson documents in her book *Out of Bedlam*, "Such a therapeutic approach to the mentally ill represents a tremendous advance over previous European techniques such as casting the mentally ill adrift on the open sea, crammed onto 'ships of fools,' or auctioning them off to the bidder who would undertake their care at the lowest cost to the public."

Today, the treatment of people with mental illness is governed by the trend toward deinstitutionalization, which has orchestrated a mass movement of the mentally ill from the state hospital to the community. This movement has been founded on the belief that the mentally ill, and also the developmentally disabled and those with other disabilities, should participate in community life to the maximum extent that their ability permits. The movement was also facilitated by the discovery in the 1950s of psychotropic drugs, which many felt would overturn the necessity for the type of custodial care the state hospitals represented.

Although constituting a tremendous advance in the treatment of mental illness, the psychotropics, such as Thorazine, were not the panacea it was hoped they would be. The majority of patients released from the state hospital flocked to boarding homes or single-room occupancies. Another segment of this population is said to comprise, depending on estimates, as much as 25% of the homeless population, and another segment has returned to their family of origin.

Reviews on the success of deinstitutionalization are mixed. Although the concepts of inclusion and participation in the life of the community are laudable, they are not always readily achieved. Many poorer communities feel that they have received a disproportionate percentage of the mentally ill, and the special needs of the new residents have created stresses on already overburdened public services. In the New Jersey seacoast towns of Asbury Park and Ocean Grove, for example, former psychiatric patients comprise as much as 10% of the population, as opposed to 2% of the general population. When residents complain that the deinstitutionalized mentally ill persons are urinating on their bushes or causing disturbances on the street because they are hallucinating, the situation leads to hostility and animosity toward the mentally ill.

The situation calls into question the rights of the individual and the community in general. In an affluent suburb of New Jersey, the community tried to have a homeless man with a history of psychiatric illness barred from the public library. It was the contention of the community that the man's poor hygiene and strange behaviors interfered with the rights of other community members to make use of and enjoy the library.

Many health care practitioners can testify to the existence of a wide range of services and quality of life that deinstitutionalization has brought about for the mentally ill. Some of the boarding homes are run and staffed by dedicated individuals who provide quality care in a home-like environment. Others are overcrowded, poorly supervised, and appear almost Dickensian in nature.

Children

Children are at a disadvantage in our culture because they are too young and inexperienced to protect and provide for themselves in our intricate web of societal needs. With only the adults who care for and interact with them to serve as their advocates, children as a special population must be given attention appropriate to their age group and developmental stage of life.

As part of a household in which caregivers come and go, children must deal with the sights and sounds of a loved one in the throes of life-threatening disease. According to Joan Hermann, MSW, ACSW, in the chapter of *Oncology Social Work: A Clinician's Guide* called "Children of Cancer Patients: Issues and Interventions," children often experience anxiety related to the impending loss of a loved one and to the next logical question — What will happen to me? Who will take care of me?

Because a child's adjustment to catastrophic illness is intimately connected to the quality of parental coping, Hermann advocates that a) children be included in honest, straightforward discussions of the illness and the treatment; b) children be given age-appropriate tasks to accommodate necessary changes in the household routine; c) children be assured that the illness is not their fault and that they will not get sick themselves; d) extended family and friends be called upon to preserve the children's normal routine as much as possible (lessons, extracurricular activities, etc.); e) the school guidance counselor and teacher be alerted to the child's situation; f) parents adhere to normal disciplinary measures and guidelines despite stress that often imposes a lack of control; and g) "family meetings" be held to help everyone cope with the stress.

The home caregiver may do well to consult with the social worker on matters pertaining to children, including daily care, funeral arrangements, bereavement follow-up, and, if necessary, placement of the child elsewhere. Children cannot be protected from the reality of illness and death, but they can learn to deal with the threat to their daily lives and their futures. Caregivers should not be afraid to interact with children, who are indeed among the most significant of significant others. Hermann writes, "Children are not that fragile and they do not suffer permanent damage because of an ill-conceived explanation or use of language" on the part of a caregiver.

Diverse Spirituality

A growing number of Americans, despite their traditional ethnic and religious groups, espouse a newfound sense of spirituality that may become a diversity issue. An individual who embraces New Age or universal thinking, as opposed to following one of the organized religions, may pose questions for caregivers about what form of spiritual services the client needs. For example, an elderly Italian woman may ask for a priest, but another woman of the same age and ethnicity may prefer a chaplain who offers eclectic points of view. Here again, the caregiver must remain non-judgmental.

Afterword on Diversity

Is it possible know all the nuances of various ethnic or racial groups, and special groups determined by age, disability, sex, religion, or special interest? Hardly. However, as health care professionals, what is possible is to cultivate an openness to new experience and an eagerness to expand our own emotional and intellectual boundaries. One sociological theory explains that most people tend to live inordinately insular lives; they are born into an ethnically, philosophically, and financially cohesive community. Throughout our lives we tend not to stray far from the community and its standard and mores. Even if we move, we tend to maintain the same types of associations: people with similar ethnic backgrounds, socioeconomic status, interests, religious affiliations. For the caregiver who becomes a guest in many a client's home and sometimes an integral part of the household's particular culture, the key is to remain open-minded and non-judgmental. If the caregiver and his or her client learn from each other and come to feel comfortable with the other's ideas and customs, the whole experience takes on an aspect of caring that extends well beyond medications, procedures, and chores.

Beyond the Melting Pot: Diversity and the Caregiver

- In matters of diversity, your clients are your primary source and they are your greatest teachers.
- Sensitivity to issues of diversity should never be used to stereotype or pigeonhole people.
- Retain your pride in your own background and life choices. Foster in others the same pride and joy you want for yourself.
- Different isn't better or worse; it is simply different.
- Home care gives you an opportunity to experience numerous cultures and ways of life that a lifetime of travel could not equal.
- In matters of diversity, openness of mind and heart is more important than knowledge.
- Always ask your clients what they preferred to be called.
- Offer in-services on cultural diversity regarding dress, grooming, food and eating customs, time consciousness, relationships, etc.
- Keep in mind that smiling and laughing may not indicate happiness or fun to one of another ethnic background; they may indicate embarrassment or discomfort. Observe, listen and be sensitive to identify the real problems.

- Assure your client confidentiality. Shame in seeking help or "losing face" in one's group may be an issue that requires attention.
- Always espouse the biopsychosocial point of view. It means "body, mind, and culture" for good reason.

Summary

- In matters of diversity, your clients are your primary source and they are your greatest teachers.

- Retain your pride in your own background and life choices. Foster in others the same pride and joy you want for yourself.

- Different isn't better or worse; it is simply different.

- Home care gives you an opportunity to experience numerous cultures and ways of life which a lifetime of travel could not equal.

- In matters of diversity, openness of mind and heart is more important than knowledge.

Chapter 4

Unique Patient/Unique Caregiver: Everyone's a Story

I don't want to belong to any club that will
accept me as a member.
Groucho Marx

The Master said, Man's very life is honesty, in that without it
he will be lucky indeed if he escapes with his life.
The Master said, To prefer it is better than only to know it.
To delight in it is better than merely to prefer it.
The Master said, To men who have risen at all above
the middling sort, one may talk of things higher yet.
But to men who are at all below the middling sort it is
useless to talk of things that are above them.
from *The Analects of Confucius*

What is it that gives us the desire to become caregivers? Is it having a much-loved mother who is a nurse, was it having our own lives changed by physical therapy, were we avid readers of *Cherry Ames, Student Nurse,* or were we devotees of the television show "Marcus Welby, MD"? For some of us, the realization comes early as a simple knowing that caregiving is what we will do for the rest of our lives. For others, the realization may come later as a recognition that this is what we *have* been doing, albeit informally, all of our lives. Certainly, there are tell-tale signs of the "Caregiver Syndrome." These are the bandagers of unsuspecting little brothers and sisters and family pets; they are the Pied Pipers of an unending stream of the lost, injured or abandoned whether of the human or animal kingdom. It has gone beyond the point of no return, when these fledgling "nurses" and "PTs" are fighting to see who gets to do the most dissecting of the fetal pig in ninth-grade biology class. (The future social workers generally don't fight much over the pig.)

Although there may be times when caring for ourselves presents a real challenge, caring for others seems as natural as breathing. Oh, there may be falls from grace when we wonder how we got involved with this anyway. We may be left wondering why we couldn't be more like cousin Louie, the computer wiz who owns a home the size of a small office building, or like our high-school friend Miriam who sells TV time and meets interesting people. Complaints about caregiving professions and paraprofessions abound: too little money, too many hours, little recognition, and hard, draining work. We are not unlike Woody Allen's joke about the two elderly Jewish ladies in the Catskills who are discussing the food. One says, "The food is lousy," and the other retorts, "Yes, and the portions are so small!" Our professions may be fraught with difficulty, yet we can't get enough. Even after taking a sabbatical to try our hand at something else, we inevitably return to caregiving like the sailor trying to ignore the call of the sea or the thespian turning his back on the footlights.

Are we admirable? At times. At our worst, we may take on the combined traits of enabler and co-dependent. At other times, we rise to the mysterious euphoria of compassion that is truly one of the most exceptional of human experiences. In any case, caregiving holds a kind of "call of the wild." We cannot ignore it. It is who we are.

What to do When Care is Rejected, Neglected or Unsuccessful

What happens when our efforts at caregiving meet with the greatest of all obstacles: patient resistance? What happens when we have a beautiful care plan, the ability to provide needed service, and the only thing we are lacking is a willing patient?

Mr. Reed is a 37-year-old librarian. While grocery shopping, Mr. Reed slipped on a small puddle of spilled juice and suffered a compound fracture. He has been out of work for six months on disability. Although the doctor feels he has made significant progress, Mr. Reed is unwilling to return to work. Generally, he appears angry. He has several lawsuits pending against the grocery and two against the doctors who treated him. In fact, Mr. Reed has a long history of litigation and seems to relish the idea of lawsuits. Several of the team members have become apprehensive about treating Mr. Reed, fearing that he will sue them, too.

Mrs. Miller is a 68-year-old widow who lives in the home in which she was born in a rural community. As a result of severe diabetes, she has lost one foot and lives primarily in a wheelchair. The care plan centered on efforts to have Mrs. Miller control her sugar intake and learn to perform her own wound care. Despite the fact that she is unfailingly pleasant and well-liked by the home care team, Mrs. Miller's sugar count remains greatly elevated, and the home health aide knows she has large boxes of "Sugar Frosted Flakes," boxes of chocolates and soft drinks in the house. When questioned about her high sugar level and the amount of sugar products in the house, Mrs. Miller seems genuinely offended and tells the nurse she keeps these items for her niece's children who visit weekly. She says she has no idea why her sugar level is so high.

In the above cases, the difficulty in treatment lies not in the conditions themselves, but rather in the personalities of the patients. How do we deal with personality traits and modes of behavior that impede treatment?

In an article in *The New England Journal of Medicine* entitled "Taking Care of the Hateful Patient," Dr. James E. Groves describes patterns of behavior typically found in difficult patients. While the title seems certainly extreme, the different personality types and behaviors are familiar to anyone who works in health care, or for that matter, operates in the real world. Groves goes on to elucidate reactions or counter-transference that these patients will often elicit in caregivers. Some of the possible responses on the part of caregivers include frustration, avoidance, aversion, or in some cases overt hostility. As Groves notes, there are serious implications to the impact that these behaviors may have on treatment, such as "there may be a 'helplessness' in the helper"; there may be an unconscious punishment of the patient; there may be self-punishment by the doctor; there may be inappropriate confrontation of the patient; and there may be a desperate attempt to avoid or to extrude the patient from the caregiving system. Although the classes of individuals described were meant to be extreme, elements of these behaviors are typically found in many interactions with patients.

The Dependent Clinger

The first category identified by Groves is that of the dependent clinger. This personality type is characterized by emotional neediness. Initially, the dependent clinger may be very appealing both to the caregiver's vanity and desire to help. Dependent clingers are often complimentary and deferential, appearing to be in awe of the caregiver's skill. Their gratitude may seem excessive, often out of proportion to the help they have received. This initial stage is very often a "honeymoon period," which is replaced by disappointment on the part of both the patient and the caregiver when the caregiver is unable to meet the dependency needs of the patient which is essentially "a bottomless pit." Although these patients may initially express gratitude at having finally found someone who can provide the help they need, as treatment progresses the patients will have ever-increasing needs for reassurance and assistance that go beyond what is reasonable to expect from the caregiver. As the dependency needs of the patient are not met, the frustration level of both patient and caregiver rises. Typically, the patient expresses disappointment and feels that his or her confidence has been misplaced.

Case Study

Cathy Williams, age 37, head of a drama department at a state university, is becoming increasingly disabled with AIDS. She is being seen by an nurse from the VNA and has expressed a number of concerns regarding her long-term living arrangement. The nurse has requested that a social worker see Ms. Williams to assist with long-term planning and provide supportive counseling.

When Greg Johnson, the agency social worker, meets Cathy Williams, he immediately likes her and feels empathy for her difficult situation. Cathy is very pleasant and expresses gratitude that this kind of help is available. Greg is somewhat awed by Cathy, an attractive and articulate woman, who lives in a beautifully restored Victorian surrounded by possessions gathered in a life of travel and theatrical involvement. Greg also feels sympathy for the many losses Cathy is presently experiencing. She has had to give up her position at the university; she is uncertain regarding her ability to cope with this illness financially; and can no longer pursue her hobbies of rock-climbing and scuba-diving. Cathy's companion of the past several years has also terminated the relationship and moved out.

After his interview with Cathy, Greg decides on a plan of care that focuses on several areas. Since Cathy has expressed a desire to remain at home, Greg explores helping her to acquire the services she needs to remain at home. Another goal of equal importance, in view of the number of losses Cathy has recently sustained, is supportive counseling. Greg's first suggestion is to have Cathy apply for live-in assistance available to the disabled through a special Medicaid program for persons with AIDS. Cathy rejects this suggestion because, she said, she values her privacy and wouldn't really want to have a stranger living with her. Cathy has also rejected the option of having her mother, who is available come to live with her. Greg begins to feel the Catch 22 of Cathy's expressed desire to remain at home and concomitant refusal to accept the means to do that.

As Greg works with Cathy, he finds a woman who materially has achieved considerable success, but for whom personal happiness has been elusive. She has been divorced twice and seems to be unable to sustain a relationship beyond a few months. Most of her friendships are professionally based, and since leaving home after college, she has had only sporadic contact with her mother and two older sisters.

As Cathy's physical condition becomes increasingly compromised, Cathy's nurse and physical therapist believe it is too dangerous for Cathy to remain in the house alone. The only assistance Cathy receives is from friends who stop over after work and an elderly neighbor who looks in on her daily. Her insurance continues to cover the expense of a home health aide who shops, does some personal care, and light housekeeping. Since Cathy has rejected the idea of live-in assistance, she is alone much of the time, and the nurse and physical therapist are afraid of her being trapped in the event of fire or caught in another emergency. They are also concerned about their own liability and that of the agency because of the questionable nature of the patient's safety. Greg receives calls from the nurse, the PT, and Cathy, asking him to find a solution. In the meantime, Cathy has also called the nursing supervisor, social work supervisor and regional health care manager complaining that no one is really helping her.

DISCUSSION

After a month in treatment, Cathy truly qualifies a "difficult patient." Team members have spent an inordinate amount of time given her physical needs, and yet feel they have accomplished little. The team holds a case conference to share perspectives and try to agree on a common course of action. During the meeting, the team members voice their frustrations and concerns and attempt to clear up any misunderstanding of what has actually taken place. Throughout the discussion, there is a common thread: the patient feels no one has adequately addressed her needs or helped. The team returns to Greg's initial assessment that Cathy needs live-in help, or that she consider a long-term care facility. The team decides that Greg and Cathy's nurse, Susan, should visit Cathy and delineate what alternatives exist.

At the meeting, Greg and Susan shared their concerns for Cathy's safety. They stated what they considered to be the best options for Cathy's care, and elicited her input. Cathy expressed her anger, fears, frustration and sadness surrounding her illness and loss of autonomy. She reluctantly agreed to having her mother move in to care for her.

Following a rocky start, Cathy and her mother seemed to resolve some of their long- standing differences. In the final stages of her illness, Cathy went on the agency's hospice program and later died. Throughout her treatment, Cathy seemed to achieve a kind of peace and equilibrium that had eluded her for much of her life.

NEED FOR DOCUMENTATION

Cathy's case brings up many issues that are important in home health care. One of the most basic issues is the need for good documentation. While clear documentation is important in any area of health care, nowhere is it more vital than in the area of home care. Without the close physical proximity afforded by the hospital or health care facility, too often team members are like "ships that pass in the night." Team members may go for days without seeing each other and rely upon the case records to give them a picture of what other team members are doing. Many clinicians feel that record-keeping is the bane of their existence, and it shows. In the worst case scenarios, it seems it is easier to reconstruct the Paleozoic period from fossils than figure out what is going on in a case from the record. Direct-care workers have many legitimate issues with record-keeping; it can be tedious, time-consuming, and cut into time one might view better spent in patient care. However, like the fossils of prehistoric times, our records are the only real proof of what we did. When there is a discrepancy as to what has transpired in a case, the record serves to corroborate the interventions that took place.

Without an accurate record, team members end up like Sherlock Holmes trying to reconstruct events from bits and fragments of information. On a basic level, written documentation gives us credit for what we do.

The most important rationale for documentation is that it provides a written history or synopsis of the care of the patient. As a history, the record keeps a detailed account of what each of the health care team members has done. It allows members of various disciplines to know the interventions of other professionals and the goals they are working toward. In addition, documentation forms the basis for a system of payment accountability for third-party payers. For instance, let's say a physical therapist has seen Mr. White, a patient whose primary insurance is Medicare, three times for an hour per visit to teach transferring. The home health care agency then submits a bill to Medicare for three hours of physical therapy for this patient. When Medicare pulls cases to assure quality control and accuracy of billing, the case record will be examined to see that in fact three hours of physical therapy were provided, that the treatment was appropriate for the patient's condition, and that the interventions are described. In the event of litigation, the case record may serve as a legal document and verify each intervention that was performed.

INFORMATION-SHARING

All too often there is not sufficient time or opportunity for team members to share information. Different schedules, heavy workloads, and rarely being in the same place at the same time can make meeting for case conferences a real challenge. In an optimum situation, the agency or organization assigns a specific time slot for case-conferencing.

Unfortunately, this may not always be the case. The detrimental effects of the failure to create opportunities to share information with other team members are readily apparent:

1. *Professional Isolation.* The geography of the home-health world makes it easy to avoid interchange with other team members. Unlike the hospital, rehab center or office, where team members see each other daily simply by coming to work, home-care workers are rarely in the office together. Often, when team members are in the office, they are occupied with picking up new cases, handing in paperwork and calling patients to make appointments and answer questions. Agencies will vary considerably in the vehicles that they create to facilitate interdisciplinary sharing. When team members do not have an opportunity to share information, it is all too easy for a misunderstanding to develop. In Cathy's case, this is easily seen by her frequent complaints to the nurse that Greg, the social worker, is not giving her any help at all. With only one part of the picture in place, Susan may assume that Cathy has in fact received no help. When Greg meets with Susan, he is able to supply some important missing information, namely that Cathy has refused several opportunities for assistance.

2. *Internal Support System.* One frequently overlooked benefit of case conferencing and information-sharing is the opportunity they create for peer support. In a well-functioning organization, frequently team members automatically develop an informal support group that mirrors many of the activities of peer support groups, such as providing a safe place to ventilate feelings of frustration, request feedback and suggest positive alternatives. It is interesting to note

that for homemakers employed by a health-care agency, supervision is seen as a vehicle for support rather than in negative hierarchical terms. "Research has shown that in-home workers perceive supervision as support, and they would like as much or more supervision than they receive," according to Salmon, 1995.

The Entitled Demander

The behavior of the entitled demander is on the opposite end of the spectrum from that of the dependent clinger. While the dependent clinger openly expresses his needs for assistance and feelings of helplessness, the entitled demander appears aggressive and very much in control.

Although both the dependent clinger and entitled demander may be acting out feelings of fear and helplessness, the outward manifestation is different. While the dependent clinger appears to be in awe of the caregiver, the entitled demander takes a disparaging view of the caregiver's capabilities. Entitled demanders seem close to hostile in their demands that caregivers give detailed accounts of their treatment and provide a justification for that course of action. The entitled demander gives the feeling that were it not for his constant vigilance, the team member could not be trusted to do the "right thing." Entitled demanders are firm believers that the squeaky wheel gets the oil. The entitled demander prides himself on being a "Ralph Nader" of life in general.

While others may be simple or gullible enough to accept people and situations as they are, entitled demanders have a "show me" attitude. They have a ready supply of stories about how their vigilance has saved them, or someone else, from some instance of incompetence or gross neglect. Essentially, they view the world as a hostile place where "survival of the fittest" reigns. As the dependent clinger may be initially endearing, arousing our protective instincts, the entitled demander evokes apprehension and irritation. All too frequently, such behavior works. People will give in or acquiesce in order to placate or avoid a scene with the entitled demander. What entitled demanders may not realize is that they have won the battle but lost the war. Although team members may give in to avoid an altercation, a residual of dislike and animosity may manifest in avoidance and a protective insulation from involvement. The entitled demander may appear in many different guises.

Case Study

At 45, Joan Hanson thought life was starting to become easier. She and her husband had raised five kids on a policeman's salary, and the tough days seemed as if they were almost over. Their oldest, Karen, 25, an elementary school teacher, was married and has a 2-year-old boy. Ellen and Marie, the next in line, had finished school and were living on their own. Pete, 21, was finishing engineering school in the spring. Only Danny, 18, in the first year of college, was still at home.

After years of diapers, yard duty, and adolescent fits, both Joan and her husband, Pete Sr., looked forward to an early retirement with a second career in a Mom-and-Pop grocery store, until Joan found she was pregnant. After the initial shock dispelled slightly, Joan, ever the survivor, tried to develop a plan. For Joan and Pete, both Catholics, abortion was out of the question. Joan fell back on the adages from her youth and tried to find the silver lining in this particular cloud. The one she was holding on to was that babies always bring happiness. Her pregnancy was difficult, with early spotting and the doctor's recommendation that she stay off her feet. When Patrick was born at seven months, he weighed four pounds and was extremely disabled with cerebral palsy. All the advice that Joan and Pete received was to put Patrick in a home.

Joan swore to herself that this would never happen and focused all her energy on Patrick. The Hansons quickly learned that the world of a special-needs child, especially 30 years ago, was and is very different. While Joan pulled closer to Patrick, Pete seemed to move further and further away, spending more time by himself and drinking more. The children, although fond of Patrick, were light years away, involved in establishing their own lives, as were Joan and Pete's friends who were starting second careers. Much of the time, it was just Joan and Patrick alone. During that time Joan came to appreciate Patrick's uniqueness in a way that the majority of people simply could not see. She saw that Patrick had a wonderful mind and unique abilities that were not readily apparent because of the short circuits caused by his brain. Joan also learned quickly that the community at large had little to offer Patrick.

Furthermore, Pete never physically left, but he withdrew more and more and was there in body only. Left on the sidelines by her family and given little help from society, Joan's life work focused on Patrick. Finding little appropriate education for those with special needs, Joan organized parent groups and became a vociferous advocate for the developmentally disabled. Joan did not accept no for an answer, and she gave many other parents the courage to do the same. Her efforts were not in vain. With the aid of many specialized learning devices and the adjustment of requirements, Patrick graduated from an excellent college with a degree in graphic design. Joan's trailblazing efforts opened worlds for Patrick and others like him. Patrick has received awards, and today, with Joan's assistance, does freelance graphic design. Patrick's accomplishments have been achieved at tremendous sacrifices on his part and that of Joan.

In the course of having succeeded in getting the best services and education available, she had given up many of the simple things—time spent with friends, hobbies, free time—and become increasingly isolated from her husband and children. When the local VNA is called in to see Patrick, Joan is poised to fight many of the battles that were relevant 30 years ago. She still sees many societal agencies in an adversarial light. She monitors the nurses' activities carefully and rejects an offer to see a social worker, saying, "They never helped me, anyway." However, she did wish to see the occupational therapist. Initially, Joan appeared critical, defensive and embittered regarding both the health care and educational systems. Based upon first reports, the team anticipated an unduly difficult case.

DISCUSSION

Joan had arrived at the role of entitled demander through a long and difficult course. The oldest child of an Irish immigrant family with six brothers and sisters, Joan couldn't remember a time when she hadn't taken care of somebody. Growing up in a poor section of Chicago, she saw life as survival of the fittest and proudly considered herself to be a "bit of a fighter." This attitude helped her raise her kids with limited finances and a husband who worked long hours. Never did this attitude seem more justified than when Patrick was born, and Joan felt every door was closed in her face. Joan's scrappy, almost pugilistic, attitude seemed to work to Patrick's benefit as person after person was forced to examine the statement, "There's nothing else we can do." Time after time, Joan believed her anger opened many doors for Patrick.

Although she felt somewhat intimidated by Joan's aggressive attitude and almost overt hostility, Karen, the nurse in charge of the case, decided to address all the patient's needs and employ a wait-and-see attitude with Joan. As Karen worked with Patrick and Joan, they agreed upon nursing visits twice a week and a referral was made for an OT evaluation. Sandy Ross, a talented and amiable occupational therapist, was assigned to the case. She quickly amazed Joan, who had much experience with physical and occupational therapists, with her creative approaches to some of the difficulties Patrick was having in working with his computer.

Gradually, Joan shared with Sandy many of difficulties and heartbreaks she endured in trying to get the best possible services for Patrick. Sandy found it a joy to work with Patrick, a bright and talented young man. Joan always remained feisty and at times confrontational, but the positive experience she and Patrick were having helped her to re-evaluate some of her hostile feelings and relax her role as entitled demander. The presence of team members helped reduce the increasing isolation she and Patrick had been experiencing and improved their quality of life. Eventually, Joan joined a local senior citizen's group that took day trips, and Patrick joined a club for persons with disabilities.

Importance of the Caregiver

When the caregiver is a gatekeeper, it is a tragic mistake to underestimate the effect the caregiver can have on the treatment a client receives. A patient with a caregiver such as Joan may suffer a number of repercussions based solely upon the caregiver's personality, such as indirect hostility, avoidance and possibly a desire to exclude the patient from the care system. Caregivers have a great deal of power in the life of the homebound patient. They function in a variety of roles relating to the patient. Some of these roles include:

1. *Gatekeepers*: On the most element level, they determine who gets to see the patient. It is generally the caregiver who arranges appointments.
2. *Care partners*: They have a tremendous impact on the implementation of the patient's care plan. Depending on the degree to which a patient is incapacitated, the caregiver may be totally responsible for dispensing medication, feeding and bathing. The quality of care the patient receives directly relates to the ability and willingness of the caregiver to perform these activities.
3. *Personal Relationship with the Patient*: There are a multitude of ways in which a caregiver may be related to a patient. The variety of relationships runs the gamut from the biological or familial, to friendships or associations of choice, to financial (those who are employed to provide care). These relationships range from those that are beneficial to those that may be negative or even abusive. Each relationship forms a unique equation based upon the personality and life situations of the caregiver and the patient. For instance, have the patient and caregiver had a long-term relationship? Has the relationship been basically positive or negative? Who seems to be the dominate person in the relationship? Have roles changed as a function of illness? Is there a history of substance abuse? Is the caregiver capable of performing his or her role physically and emotionally?

Primacy of Patient Care

In a case like this, it would be easy for Patrick to get lost in the shuffle. With a caregiver such as Joan, who seems hostile and aggressive and very much the gatekeeper, it would be easy for the health-care team to expend all its energy just dealing with Joan. Of course, this would eliminate the most important team member, Patrick. Here the ability of the team member to deal with the family dynamic between Patrick and Joan, an entitled demander, opened the door for Patrick to receive the care he needed. Additionally, what contributed to the successful resolution was the ability of team members to see beyond the limitations of Joan's aggressive and almost hostile behavior, and recognize that much of this was residual behavior that had once been necessary in order for Joan to give Patrick the very best. When staff members didn't respond in a defensive manner, it opened the door to a more productive relationship. By engaging in a dialogue, Joan, who initially acted so intimidating, became, in fact, an excellent care-partner who contributed to an improvement in Patrick's quality of life and helped arrive at ingenious solutions to the problems inherent to Patrick's condition.

Self-Destructive Deniers

Self-destructive deniers are distinguished by their blatant disregard for even minimal precautions. These are the drinkers with liver involvement who know one more drink may kill them and don't even slow down. They are the smokers who have lung cancer and crawl to the bathroom for a cigarette, or the person with diabetes who has lost a limb and remains a patron of fast-food places and doughnut shops. They seem beyond fear. They are the patients from hell and a caregiver's worst nightmare. They do not emerge with the overt hostility of the entitled demander or the insatiable demands of the dependent clinger. Yet they defeat every effort at care. In fact, they ask for nothing.

However, they fly in the face of everything a caregiver holds sacred. In "Taking Care of the Hateful Patient," Groves distinguishes between self- destructive deniers and major deniers: self-destructive deniers are often almost aggressive in their lack of care, while major deniers suffer more from benign neglect. Major deniers may be stoic to the point of viewing self-care as a self-indulgence. Often major deniers are too busy caring for others to care for themselves. Unlike the self-destructive deniers, who seem bent upon destroying themselves, major deniers may respond to gentle prodding. Unless self-destructive deniers have a major epiphany, it is unlikely that they will be swayed from their ill-fated course of action.

There is a bizarre quality to the actions of self-destructive deniers as they smoke with tracheotomies, use prescribed drugs in dangerous combinations, and drink until they hallucinate. While initially caregivers may see this patient as a challenge and feel that they will be the ones to reach him or her, the stage is generally short-lived. Caregivers will quickly come to feel that their efforts have little, if any, effect and may come to believe their time would be better spent with other patients. A possible negative reaction to the self-destructive denier may even be an attempt to exclude the patient from the service delivery system. For example, the efforts of the emergency staff of a large metropolitan hospital discontinued services to a patient with chronic alcoholism by instructing him that when he was on a binge, he was to stay on a certain side of the street that would place him in another hospital's jurisdiction.

Case Study

At 42, Dudley Ashton had been in alcohol rehabs more times than he could count. He had even followed a circuit known to hard-core alcoholics in which he spent the cold months in the warmer climates like Florida and worked his way north for the summer. He knew where the Salvation Armies were in each state, and he had been a frequent visitor. In the days before homelessness had reached today's proportions, Dudley spent most of his adult life homeless. Since age 18, his longest employment was a job he held for three months, in which he was being considered for management training. One day Dudley did not return from lunch. He was on the road again. He lived in abandoned cars, burned-out buildings and under bridges and was a bona fide citizen of a kind of American Third World. Dudley knew how to survive. He knew where to go when his clothes were threadbare and his shoes had holes.

He said he knew every soup kitchen on the Eastern Seaboard. Dudley drank and smoked as much as he could. His most distinguishing feature was his personality. Unremarkable for his height, weight and physical countenance, Dudley had one truly remarkable characteristic: an astonishing ability to get along with people. It didn't matter what a person's circumstances—a neurosurgeon or a person sleeping in a train station—Dudley could put someone completely at ease. He attributed his ease with people to his early years being raised in a brothel, where his mother was the madam and all his aunts worked. Dudley felt he had seen all manner of people and was shocked by little. Rather than leaving him insensitive or aggressive, it made him strangely accepting of people, whatever their circumstances.

But years of living out had taken their toll on Dudley's health. Although his chronological age was 44, his physiological age was that of a much older man. Dudley would laugh and say, "If you lived my life, you'd have a lot wrong with you, too." In addition to a myriad of complaints ranging from rheumatism to fallen arches, Dudley became concerned when his life-long "smoker's cough" became increasingly persistent and he began to cough up blood. The nurse at the alcohol rehab where Dudley was an inpatient was very concerned and sent him to the local hospital for a work-up. The first set of x-rays revealed the whole story.

Dudley had advanced lung cancer. When given the dim prognosis, he was somewhat stunned but took it stoically. But when the physician suggested courses of radiation and chemotherapy, Dudley refused. It appeared that Dudley's doctors and nurses and the staff from the rehab were having a tough time accepting Dudley's decision not to pursue treatment.

DISCUSSION

Self-destructive deniers pose difficult problems for the health caregiver. Virtually all their behaviors undermine what the health caregiver strives to achieve. Self-destructive deniers efforts' at self-destruction are always far ahead of the caregiver's interventions. Because they leave such little chance of even minimal success, the self-destructive deniers engender negativity such as impotence, depression, anger and hostility in caregivers. The behavior of self-destructive deniers is so extreme that, if it were directed at another person, it would probably be considered criminal. Groves explains: "They may represent a chronic form of suicidal behavior; often they let themselves die."

Self-destructive deniers may be the ultimate lesson in professional humility. Here, we can lead the horse to water and not only will he not drink, but we may very likely get kicked in the process. The determination to stay ill seems to defy all measures of knowledge and intervention. While certainly one of the most difficult patients to deal with, self-destructive deniers offer opportunities for professional growth.

A patient with this type of behavior forces us to intensely examine our own motivations. Some of the questions we are led to include: When have we done enough for a patient? Can we accept a patient's decision to accept treatment? How will this alter our feelings about the patient?

The twelve-step programs can be very helpful in teaching us to deal with this kind of behavior. Fundamental to these programs for the patient with an addiction is admission that the person is powerless against his or her addiction. Similarly, caregivers need to recognize that we are powerless to change another human being. We can give our patients the tools and benefits of skill and expertise, but we cannot make decisions for them.

Another lesson that we may take from our friends in twelve-step programs is that our efforts may not be as lost as we think. There are cases that do turn around. Often when seemingly unalterably self-destructive individuals change, they report a cumulative effect of interventions and efforts to help.

Implications for Practice

CLIENT SELF-DETERMINATION

One of the most glaring issues raised by cases like Dudley's is the fact that we are not always able to alter our patients' behavior. With the exception of activities that are overtly harmful to oneself or another, as caregivers, we are powerless to stop our patients from a self-destructive course of action. As caregivers, the inability to change overtly self-destructive behaviors may be one of the most difficult issues we have to face.

Manipulative Help-Rejecters

Dependent Clinger

Frank Smith, a retired accountant, has been sent home after a massive heart attack. He lives with his wife, Josephine, in an affluent neighborhood on the outskirts of town. The couple's three children all live out of state. Josephine has never gotten her driver's license, and Frank has always taken her shopping. Josephine requests that the home health aide, Sharon, a 25-year old single parent, take her grocery shopping. Sharon says she is prohibited from driving a patient's vehicle.

During the week she was assigned to Mr. Smith, Sharon became quite fond of both Frank and Josephine. Josephine tells Sharon that she is really in a bind and has no other way of getting to the grocery store. She asks Sharon to take her by using Frank's car and tells her not to worry, "No one will find out." Unfortunately, Sharon gets into a minor accident with Frank's expensive car, and Josephine is taken to the hospital complaining of whiplash. Josephine calls the VNA to see if it will assume responsibility for the accident.

DISCUSSION

Whatever form manipulative behavior takes, be it aggressively demanding, or heart-wrenchingly needy, there is generally a common denominator in the goals it intends to achieve. The purpose is generally to get the team member to do something he or she is not comfortable doing. How do we separate a legitimate request from an inappropriate or manipulative one? While not terribly scientific, an almost surefire gauge of manipulative behavior is the caregiver's own feelings. Most appropriate requests by patients or caregivers are easily handled and arouse no anxiety. However, a request that makes us uncomfortable is likely to contain a component of manipulation. Most of us learn to deal with manipulative behavior by being exposed to it, and probably succumbing more often than we would like to admit. The effects of allowing ourselves to be manipulated can range from simple annoyance to compromising ourselves and our organization professionally. Take, for instance, the case of Sharon's using the patient's car. Here, the agency was faced with a possible lawsuit, and the home health aide came close to being fired. One of the best defenses against manipulative behavior is to give yourself space to deal with it. In very few circumstances are we obligated to give someone an immediate answer. We can give ourselves time by simply telling the patient or caregiver we will "get back to them on that."

Virginia Astir developed a model for common verbal behavior patterns that is helpful in identifying some of the ways people use communication styles to respond to their environment. Familiarity with these styles of communication can provide strategies for some of the resistance encountered in treating patients. The styles of communication Satir identified include the following.

The Placater

In this style of communication, the person always seeks to accommodate. Primarily coming from a vantage of fear of rejection and hostility, the placater tries to appease others. He or she has an aversion to hostility and aggression and a desire to maintain pleasant relations. What the placater says does not necessarily reflect what he feels or what he is doing in reality. A placater may be difficult to confront because of the tendency to deny disagreement. In the case of Mrs. Miller, she is unwilling to admit that she is not complying with the treatment plan.

Another category noted by Groves is that of the help-rejecter. Here the patient is pessimistic regarding the success of any intervention or plan or care. Inevitably, attempts at treatment meet with failure. This type of behavior is sometimes viewed as a subconscious attempt to prolong indefinitely the helping relationship. A help-rejecting patient will very often have a long history of medical intervention that provides no relief. The frustration level of caregivers can rise quickly as they come to realize that their interventions seem doomed to failure.

The Manipulative Patient

Although not included in Groves' description of the difficult patient, the home health team member is particularly vulnerable to manipulations on the part of the home care patient. Any one of the personality types described can engage in manipulative behavior, and the personality type of the person involved will simply dictate the form of manipulation. Two factors increase the likelihood of manipulation in the home care setting: first, the patient is on his or her own turf, and in essence, the home-care worker is a guest in the patient's home. This may equalize the patient and caregiver in terms of power. Second, the caregiver is geographically isolated from other team members and their support system.

Entitled-Demander

Mr. Harris is caring for his 57-year-old wife who has had a severe CVA. Following her stroke and hospitalization, his private insurance company authorized a number of home health services including skilled nursing, physical therapy, home health aide assistance and social work. After six weeks of care, Mrs. Harris' condition is deemed chronic and no longer subject to remediation, and the insurance company no longer authorized home services. Mr. Harris is irate and telephones the home health agency, demanding it continue to provide services because he is unable to care for Mrs. Harris. When he is informed that the home health agency is no longer being reimbursed, he demands that service be continued and says he personally knows of a number of cases in which patients have continued to receive care. He threatens to go to the local newspaper and the mayor.

The Blamer

Here the primary strategy is one of attack. The blamer tends to externalize blame. He or she freely rattles off a litany of complaints. A blamer can be painful for a well-motivated caregiver to deal with because he tends to personalize the attacks, which usually contain the component of "If only you had....(been more sensitive, done your job better, acted more quickly, etc.)." Blamers often feel that by putting the other person on the defensive, they become more powerful. They can become very hostile when they do not achieve what they want. Attempts to appease a blamer are rarely successful because blamers need to find a reason to be upset. As Suzette Haden Elgin, a psycholinguist who applies Satir's principles in her book, *The Gentle Art of Verbal Self-Defense,* writes, "When two blamers talk to each other, it is not a dead end, as it is with two placaters. It is a broad and rapid road to a screaming match, nasty in every way."

Blamers can be very frustrating to deal with because they are "bottomless pits" for whom nothing will ever be good enough. They are expert fault-finders. It is a small wonder that Mr. Reed has a series of lawsuits behind him. He would be deeply disappointed if he couldn't find fault somewhere.

The Leveler

The leveler is someone who gives what he believes to be an honest assessment of the situation both intellectually and emotionally. In many ways, to be able to communicate on the subject of the leveler is enormously positive personally and professionally. In this type of communication, the leveler is conveying his or her perception without blaming or fearing the disapproval of others. The leveler's style requires less decoding, which can be a very difficult job. Here we don't have to get past the blaming and placating styles of Mrs. Miller and Mr. Reed to give levelers the help they need.

A "true leveler" is often the easiest style to maneuver. However, a "false leveler," as Suzette Haden Elgin notes, can be the most difficult. A false leveler will appear to be sharing his feelings and judgments, while he is really blaming or placating or distracting (see *The Distracter*) in the guise of being up front.

The Computer

The person who employs this type of communication is an arsenal of information. He or she is the "Trivial Pursuit" master of the real world. Excellent historians, computers' reports take on a clinical quality we could almost envy. It is rare for them to have any difficulty in remembering when symptoms began, what the diagnosis was, or how they were treated. Strangely missing in any of their descriptions, however, are any emotional references. Their wealth of information, and at times obsession with detail, are very often a defense against allowing themselves to feel. Information is seen as a tool with which to master their worlds. Often, computers seem to miss the forest for the trees.

Mr. Walsh is a recently retired executive whose wife of 40 years is dying of breast cancer. He grew up a poor child on the streets of New York's Lower East Side. When he went to work in the mail room of a large company, he had little to recommend him other than his eighth-grade education. What Mr. Walsh did possess was an astonishing memory for details and an affable disposition. His ability to retain information made him stand out, and he rose quickly in the company's ranks. In the days before computers, Mr. Walsh was the company "computer."

As he cares for Mrs. Walsh, the health care team is amazed by Mr. Walsh's organization. He knows exactly who is coming and when, understands all his wife's medications, and turns her every few hours. But the emotional element is undetectable. Mr. Walsh seems to become uncomfortable when a caregiver alludes to his own pain. The fact that Mr. Walsh is losing his childhood sweetheart, the mother of their five children and his golfing buddy is something he is either unable or unwilling to discuss.

The Distracter

This type of communicator is possibly the most difficult to pin down. Although you may not agree with the basic premise of the placater, blamer or computer, their arguments seem cohesive. You can follow their line of reasoning. For example, if you can momentarily concur with the computer that details rule the world, then being organized will certainly give you a leg up on everyone else. If you can agree with the blame that the physician should have prescribed another type of chemotherapy, then that error will be the root of their pain. On the other hand, the distracters bring in so much that is extraneous—a flight of ideas—that it is difficult to determine what their argument is or where they are coming from.

Mrs. Richards, the mother of three young children, is being treated for emphysema. It is difficult to get her to commit to a time for home health visits. The children need to be taken to school, and then, of course, they have after-school activities. Mr. Richards' family from Chicago will be visiting soon. Mrs. Richards never really had health problems before, and she hasn't really discussed them with the children. Of course, she will soon.

Chapter 4

What Do These Divergent Styles Mean to Us as Caregivers?

Understanding the different styles of communications can help make us more objective and less reactive in our work with patients. It can also help to suggest various strategies to deal with patterns that place obstacles in the path toward the well-being of our patients. It can also help to examine our own patterns of behaviors to see how they are helping or hindering our interactions with patients. Identifying the patterns as belonging to the patient helps establish a boundary where we feel less pulled in and freer to respond from our own point of view.

This knowledge also helps us disengage from the patient's personal issues. Getting caught up in the patient's problems tends to make them our own, which we then feel obligated to resolve. Rarely is this successful. More frequently, it leads to a cycle of frustration and failure. As we try to solve the blamer's complaints, we will be frustrated to find that more complaints emerge. As we enter the flaky world of the distracter, our own treatment focus may be lost. But by looking as objectively as possible at the client's behavior, we are better able to determine how we should behave. It frees us to develop more of the leveler in our own behavior.

Examining our own behavior can help us to see where we need to grow in our professional lives. If we tend to placate, we can sense the frustration of the patient whose concerns get minimized. We can empathize with the anxiety of the patient awaiting blood-test results and in dealing with the distracter whose conversation races from her son's Little League scores to the weather before she gets down to business. We can feel the sense of anger of the patient dealing with the blamer who smugly tells him, "If only you did what you were supposed to do, you'd be feeling better."

Appreciate, above all, the emotional clarity of telling a patient, "This is how I see your situation, and this is what I think you need to do." Then step back to allow the client to make his or her own decisions. In sum, the successful caregiver pursues the issues at hand, accepts the client's response style, and compassionately helps the client stay on track.

Patient Strengths

Regardless of our problems, all too frequently we seem intent upon focusing on problems or disabilities as opposed to focusing on strengths. Whatever our patients' condition or disability, we may see only that we will be neglecting important components that will contribute to their recovery. This is the perennial issue of whether the cup is half-full or half-empty. This does not take into account those who see it as three-quarters-full or three quarters-empty. It is all a matter of perception.

If we look at a 75-year-old man with chronic obstructive pulmonary disease (COPD) from the point of pathology and see only a frail man with a few months to live, we lose sight of the much broader and more important picture. We fail to see the young man who supported a widowed mother, brothers and sisters, the railroad man who worked at a physically demanding job for nearly 50 years, the husband and father who lost a home during the Depression and went out and started over. We fail to see an indomitable spirit.

The same is true if we look at a patient with AIDS and see only the tragedy, rather than a mother who rises above tragedy to plan Christmas for her family. All patients are survivors. They would not be here if they were not. To hear the litany of losses of many of our patients would make our knees buckle. One of the most productive ways we can work with clients is to focus not on their weaknesses, but on their strengths.

In the article "How to Interview for Client Strengths" in *Social Work,* Peter DeJong and Scott Miller view the strengths perspective as resting on five assumptions:

1. In spite of difficulties and problems, all people and environments possess strengths that can be employed to improve clients' lives.
2. Clients are motivated by a recognition of strengths as defined by the clients.
3. Discovering strengths is a process of exploration by the client and the practitioner.
4. Focusing on client's strengths helps to neutralize a "blame the victim" stance and engenders respect for client coping skills in difficult environments.
5. Broadens the practitioner's perspective to incorporate the idea that all environments contain resources.

Case History

Jane Winston is a 35-year-old patient with AIDS. Jane contracted HIV from her husband, Steve, 38, who has a history of intravenous drug use and drug-related convictions. Jane was diagnosed 2 years ago. Steve and Jane have been married for 18 years and have two sons, Steve Jr., 17, and Ryan, 6. Jane has been conscientious about complying with her medical regime and hospital appointments. She has also tried to assist

Steve. Jane continues to work part-time at a local department store. Both she and Steve are being seen by the nurse and social worker from the local VNA under a special Medicaid program for persons with AIDS. Both the nurse and social worker strongly suspect that Steve is still engaging in drug use.

Jane's concerns center on making the most of Steve's health and her own. She is also concerned with getting help in taking care of medical bills which predate her special Medicaid program, and she would like assistance in gaining Section 8 housing since, as she becomes increasingly ill, her earning ability will decrease. Jane has resisted efforts to get her to join a support group, saying she is not a "joiner."

DISCUSSION

If we take this case from a perspective of illness or pathology, we may see Jane as extremely co-dependent and lacking in self-esteem, with minimal education. There is much evidence to support this assessment, beginning with her childhood when she functioned as a parental child in a home in which both parents were alcoholic, and she was often left in charge of the younger children when the parents were drinking. The pattern continued as Jane grew up to marry a man who is emotionally immature and has problems with substance abuse. Here again, Jane continues in the role she learned in childhood, that of "holding everything together." There is also Jane's perception of herself as "the strong one."

Perhaps the first thing we need to realize is that Jane is not seeking psychotherapy or counseling. Her concerns are concrete: she is invested in gaining for herself and her husband the best quality of life and care available, and she wants to develop a long-term plan to address their medical and financial needs. Previous experiences with team members have shown Jane to be an excellent caregiver whose quality of care accounts for the couple's optimal state of health given their disease. As team members are able to rally with Jane around her issues—the nurse monitoring their health and medication, the dietitian recommending an appropriate diet, the social worker's clearing up old medical bills and trying to get Section 8 housing—the case goes extremely well.

Summary

- Meeting patients at a time of illness or crisis may often give a skewed picture of both the patient and support system.

- We need to make the most of limited time we have with patients to make important assessments.

- Be aware that the information you have may only be the tip of the iceberg.

- Go beyond the superficial in relating to your patients.

- The more patients open up, the greater your ability to provide care.

- It is difficult to assess the negative effects of narrowmindedness in health care, but it may link with possible recurrence of or failure to prevent illness, and lack of appropriate planning.

- Telling one's story is therapeutic.

- While certain patients may capture our hearts, others will be pleasant encounters, and some will drive us up the wall. They are all entitled to the same high level of care.

- Patients use their styles because they work, not to make your life a misery. Learn what styles are particularly difficult for you to deal with.

- Move away from a reactive stance. Learn Murray Bowen's technique of the "I" statement.

- Compare your feelings with those of other team members. It serves as a reality check.

Never the "Lone Ranger": The Health-Care Team

It is through love that we elevate ourselves. And it is through love for others that we assist others to elevate themselves.
M. Scott Peck, "Meditations From the Road"

... The union of hearts, the union of hands. . .
George Pope Morris, "The Flag of our Union"

On Grenada, the largest of the Grenadine Islands in the Caribbean, a person who desires to build a house catches the ear and sympathy of fellow Grenadians. They all gather to help in a house-building party called a "maroon." The men make short work of the wood and supplies; the women provide food and drink. Everyone is important in the project.

It is amazing what can happen in a health-care "maroon," when a patient has the benefit of several astute minds concentrating on his or her well-being, and many talented hands that perform treatments, procedures and other tasks designed to bolster the patient's body and attitude. In order to do their best work independently and as a team, health caregivers need to know who the others are, their roles, and the most effective means of interaction and cooperation. Here the professionals and non-professionals are outlined in the interest of their common goal: to help improve the patient's physical and emotional state.

The Physician (MD or DO)

A person with a baccalaureate degree, usually in a biological science or "pre-med" studies, and several more years of graduate study leading to the degree of Medical Doctor (MD) or Doctor of Osteopathy (DO), and who is thereafter licensed to practice medicine and surgery. Some physicians specialize in family practice (also called general practitioners), pediatrics, surgery, ophthalmology, radiology, oncology, cardiology, obstetrics and gynecology, otolaryngology, urology, neurology, psychiatry and other branches of medicine. The physician makes diagnoses, orders medications and treatments, and directs and coordinates the patient's care.

The Physiatrist (MD or DO)

A medical doctor (MD or DO) who specializes in physical medicine and rehabilitation, a medical specialty that focuses on helping patients overcome disabilities or impairments that occur as a result of illness such as strokes or wasting diseases, or trauma, particularly injury to the joints and muscles. The physiatrist establishes a rehabilitation program and coordinates and supervises the therapists who administer the treatments.

The Nurse Practitioner (NP)

A registered nurse with a master's degree in family practice, gerontology or other specialty who treats chronic stable or minor acute conditions. Many nurse practitioners are permitted to prescribe medications and treatments for these conditions. Some nurse practitioners have their own offices and work under the auspices of a physician.

The Registered Nurse (RN)

A person who has had 2 or more years of theoretical and clinical training and who must pass state licensing examinations in order to practice nursing. Many registered nurses now have a bachelor's and master's degree. They make nursing assessments and diagnoses (non-medical), monitor patients' vital signs, administer medications according to the physician's orders, teach patients self-care, and educate them on matters of illness, wellness and prevention. Nurses may be certified through additional training to set up intravenous lines, work in the operating room, assist at births, administer anesthesia and perform other tasks that require theoretical and scientific knowledge.

The Practical or Vocational Nurse (LPN or LVN)

A person who has 1 year or more of less technical training than that of a registered nurse, but who has passed a state licensing examination. LPNs and LVNs are supervised by physicians and RNs.

The Nurse's Aide

A hospital or home-care employee who helps patients with personal hygiene, feeding, and transferring from one location to another, such as from the bed to the bathroom or the chair to the bed. Some home health nurse's aides are allowed to give medications under the supervision of the patient's family and physician, and assist in treatments given by professional caregivers.

The Medical Social Worker (MSW)

The medical social worker, who holds a master's degree and various licenses acquired through passing post-graduate state examinations, helps patients in a number of ways, including psychological counseling and arranging post-hospital care services and medical financing.

The Psychiatric Social Worker

The psychiatric social worker specializes in emotional and psychological counseling.

The Physical Therapist (PT)

A college-educated person trained and licensed to administer physical therapy, which is the treatment of trauma or disorders that respond to physical exercise, heat, cold, ultrasound, diathermy, hydrotherapy, phototherapy and various electrical currents. Physical therapy also focuses on preventive measures against joint stiffness, muscle atrophy or weakness, pain, inflammation, spasms and motor-coordination problems.

The Physical Therapy Assistant (PTA)

A professional assistant (some states require licensure) to the PT who works both independently and tests, evaluates, observes and helps patients during therapeutic treatment sessions. The PTA may also train patients in the use of rehabilitative devices such as splints, braces, and prostheses and report the patient's progress to the PT. Some PTAs administer treatments according to the orders of the physical therapist. The PTA must complete a 2-year associate's degree program.

The Dietitian (RD) or Nutritionist

A college-educated person, frequently with a master's degree, who specializes in dietetics, which is the science of applying nutritional principles and data to the diets of sick and healthy persons. The registered dietitian also teaches nutrition to patients in order to prevent disease processes and ill-being.

The Respiratory Therapist (RT)

A college-educated, licensed person who administers respiratory care and treatments, including breathing exercises and instruction in the use of devices such as ventilators, oxygen tents, etc., according to the physician's orders. Respiratory therapy involves evaluation, diagnosis, treatment, control and rehabilitation of life-threatening airway disturbances, particularly acute breathing problems as a result of head injury, drowning, drug toxicity, cardiac failure, stroke, shock and diseases such as asthma and emphysema. There are three classifications of respiratory-therapy careers: respiratory therapist, respiratory therapy technician, and respiratory therapy aide. The technician and the aide work under the auspices of the therapist.

The Speech Therapist (ST) and Audiologist

College-educated and licensed specialist in speech and language disorders caused by stroke, laryngectomy or a particular disease process that impairs one's ability to communicate. The audiologist detects hearing impairment and disorders and assists individuals with appropriate interventions.

The Occupational Therapist (OT)

A college-educated, licensed specialist concerned with an impaired individual's ability to perform activities of daily living, which usually involve motor coordination, and his psychosocial skills that may have been impaired by a physical or mental disorder. The OT uses procedures based on self-care, educational, social and vocational concepts and teaches the use of adaptive devices to help clients dress, eat, reach for things, etc.

The Occupational Therapy Assistant (OTA)

A professional assistant to the occupational therapist (see Chapter 6), who provides care and treatment under the auspices of an OT. The Certified OTA, or COTA, holds an associate degree and has passed a national certification examination given by the American Occupational Therapy Association Certification Board. The COTA may also have had 2 years of experience as an OTA and passed a proficiency exam sponsored by the US Public Health Service before December 13, 1977.

The Pharmacist (RPh)

College-educated, licensed specialist in the science of drugs who prepares and dispenses prescriptions and over-the-counter drugs. The pharmacist often serves as a consultant to physicians, nurses and the public on the selection, correct dosage and effects of drugs.

The Chiropractor or Chiropractic Physician (DC)

A person with a doctoral degree in chiropractic, a branch of the healing arts that emphasizes spinal mechanics and neurological, muscular and vascular interactions in the event of illness. Chiropractors do not prescribe drugs or perform surgery; they perform physio-therapeutic techniques including spinal adjustment. There are several schools of chiropractic.

The Dentist (DDS)

Doctors of dental surgery, who diagnose and treat oral diseases and disorders, fill cavities, extract teeth, provide dentures and cosmetic tooth repair, and teach preventive care of the teeth and gums.

The Podiatrist (DPM)

Formerly called chiropodist, the doctor of podiatric medicine diagnoses and treats foot diseases, injuries and deformities. The podiatrist may use surgery, medication, and orthotics (devices that support the foot in such a way as to rearrange or correct the weight bearing parts of the foot). In the case of severe foot and leg disease, the podiatrist refers the patient to a physician (MD).

The Clergy or Chaplain

Usually a college-educated person, frequently with a Doctor of Divinity degree, who specializes in helping people deal with spiritual and emotional problems. Many priests, nuns, ministers, rabbis and other spiritual workers also provide psychological counseling.

The Family Team

According to psychotherapist Stephanie Matthews Simonton, in her book *The Healing Family: The Simonton Approach for Families Facing Illness* (Bantam, 1984), the family members and the patient form a crucial support system for each other. In the family team, she writes, there is not equal freedom and decision-making power, but rather clear adult leadership and an appropriate division of responsibility. Simonton advocates individual autonomy, "which means each member is encouraged to be responsible for himself, to think freely and express his own opinions. Without this respect for individuality, the family cannot operate well as a team."

In the case of catastrophic illness, the patient needs to maintain his autonomy instead of becoming passive, and the family may need to learn not to overprotect the patient. In order to heal, he must mobilize his personal resources. Each family member must now openly state his needs—not a typical process in most families—so they can become "a healing family." Among the principles Simonton sets forth for the healing family are:

1. The patient is the captain of the team. For example, if the patient is a woman who always handled the finances, she may feel comforted to know who will pay the bills and balance the accounts. A woman who was a homemaker may take great comfort in knowing how the laundry will get done, etc. The patient is to be included in all possible decisions to bolster his or her sense of control and as a way to encourage hope.

2. The family will find a way to meet each member's important needs. There is no reason to set aside everyone's life in deference to the ill person. Furthermore, it may be harmful to do so. Be creative; there's always *some* way.

3. Give the patient an opportunity to rest and relieve anxiety. Delegate some tasks to friends and relatives, such as taking Susie to piano lessons.

4. Keep lines of communication open. You are allowed to have an opposing opinion and to express it.

5. Share rather than conceal feelings. If possible, seek a therapist or counselor. Illness breeds many personal, difficult issues, and it is okay to ask for help.

6. Let the little ones help. They can rub the patient's back, feet or hands, or play cards with the patient, etc.

7. The older children should not only help, but in the process learn to be considerate of others.

8. Develop outside support systems; don't overwork the work ethic.

9. Encourage family members (including the patient if he or she is able) to exercise.

10. If the patient is a child, remember that being different from peers is the most difficult situation. But the child can be encouraged and supported into being comfortable with himself. Children need unconditional love and acceptance.

Caregivers

How do we become caregivers? Unlike the team member, caregivers generally do not choose caregiving. It is chosen by circumstances beyond their control. Unlike the health professionals, they do not arrive at caregiving by selecting a course of study or filling out a job application. Caregivers are there simply by virtue of being someone's son, daughter, wife, husband, neighbor, lover or friend. In a strange way, caregiving may be part of the admission price of being human. Oddly enough, it may also be part of the reward. Most probably they would not elect it. Unlike the team member, the caregiver's formal preparation is probably nil. Caregivers may have been caring for others as long as they can remember, or it may be an uncomfortably new role. Whether experienced or inexperienced, it is a role that incorporates a spectrum of emotions—anxiety, fatigue, resentment, guilt, and, it is hoped, a good deal of personal satisfaction.

Effects of Caregiving

Role Reversal

Emblematic of the difficulty encountered by unprepared caregivers is the old adage "One mother can care for 10 children, but 10 children can't care for one mother." A common scenario one encounters in health care is that the patient had been the primary caregiver in the family, and, in addition to the trauma of the patient's illness, the family is often at a loss as to how the role will be filled.

Take, for example, the case of Mrs. Meyers, who has been married for 50 years and during that time filled a traditional role: homemaker, nurturer and community representative. Mr. Meyers, a truck driver, was the breadwinner and responsible for meeting the family's basic needs. This arrangement was acceptable to both of them. However, when Mrs. Meyers had a massive CVA and was released from the hospital, her husband panicked. He had never had to boil an egg, and suddenly he was faced with caring for a totally disabled person. The Meyers' have three adult children, all of whom live out of state.

Although Mr. Meyers is somewhat intimidated by assuming his new role, he is willing to learn. As he says, "I survived the Depression, I'll survive this." When the visiting nurse arrived on the first day, she and Mr. Meyers discussed Mrs. Meyers' care needs and how they can best be met.

Fatigue

As Golodetz describes, the caregiver has none of the protection of the employed person. For the caregiver, it is a 24-hour job that many times is physically demanding and emotionally stressful. Add to this the fact that many caregivers are elderly and frail themselves. The help they receive is often minimal under the guidelines of Medicare and insurance policies. Many caregivers may be the sole support of the patient and receive little or no help from relatives, neighbors or community programs. The caregiving regime may interfere with established patterns of the caregiver, such as the need to awaken in the middle of the night to dispense medication. A patient may be restless and keeps the caregiver awake, which represents a reversal of the patient's sleep patterns.

Mrs. Walsh, a 73-year-old caregiver, was trying to help her 80-year-old husband in the shower after he was released from the hospital. He had had a heart attack. They both fell in the shower and remained there until their daughter came to visit 12 hours later.

Isolation

The demands of caregiving can often lead to isolation. Unless the patient has maintained a fair amount of independence, the caregiver is likely to be on call 24 hours a day. With such a demanding situation, often the first thing to be sacrificed is the caregiver's necessary and leisure activities. Caregivers also frequently report feeling that no one understands what they are going through. Suddenly, their lives revolve completely around the needs of the patient.

Depression

All the factors mentioned—fatigue, isolation, role-overload and grief—can combine to lead to a situational depression on the part of the caregiver. In addition, there is the element of uncertainty. Even a highly skilled assessment and prognosis can only give the parameters of what one may expect in a situation. For each case that falls within these parameters, there are also others that elude the probabilities. For people who are trying to plan their lives, uncertainty can also translate as seeing no light at the end of the tunnel. The perceived inability to control one's life can lead to resentment, which in turn may lead to guilt for being less altruistic than one would like to be. All of these emotional issues left unaddressed can result in situational depression.

Resources to be Offered to Caregivers

Emotional Support

Possibly the greatest resource we can offer the caregiver is emotional support. A study done in the 1960s in England on the satisfaction of homemakers related a lack of satisfaction to the absence of concrete and quantifiable reinforcement contributed to a lack of value in the role of homemaker. The study contrasted the role of the homemaker to that of the employed person, who operates under highly defined parameters that determine what he will get paid, how he or she will advance, and that specify the responsibilities of the job. In many ways, the homemaker's situation parallels that of the caregiver, because it is without the concrete reinforcements of employment.

Chapter 5

1. Establish a relationship with the caregiver(s).
2. Be empathetic with the difficulties of the caregiver role.
3. Respect the caregiver's boundaries.
4. Allow caregivers to ventilate their concerns and hardships.
5. Praise their efforts.
6. Encourage them to meet their own needs.

Referral to Community Resources

Referral to community resources may end up being as much a benefit to the caregiver as it is to the patient. Whatever services are provided—"Meals on Wheels, transportation, etc.—inevitably they will free up time for the caregiver. Here, too, the volunteer is an invaluable resource to both patient and caregiver. Something as simple as getting a haircut may become an obstacle for a caregiver.

Mr. Samuels, a dapper man in his eighties, was providing excellent care for his wife who suffers from Alzheimer's disease. Although a home health aide has been assigned to come twice a week, Mr. Samuels has used that time to run errands and has been reluctant to get a haircut, since the shop is on the other side of town. The nurse suggested a volunteer who can once a week give Mr. Samuels much-needed free time. The volunteer worked out beautifully; the caregiver can now attend in some small way to his own needs.

RESOURCES FOR THE CAREGIVER

Among the important resources for caregivers are family supports, respite care and support groups. By encouraging caregivers to accept help from family members, you increase the likelihood that they will not be overwhelmed by the stresses of caregiving. Making the caregiver aware of the respite programs that exist in the community increases their alternatives. Frequently these programs have long waiting lists, so it is helpful to start the process early.

Another avenue that is a tremendous resource for caregivers is the various support groups that are available. A great many hospitals offer these groups as a community service. The types of groups run the gamut from general caregivers' groups to groups specifically designed for caregivers of persons with Alzheimer's, cancer or other catastrophic illness. Groups vary, but they typically offer information and emotional support. They tend to decrease caregiver isolation socially and emotionally because they bring caregivers into contact with others in a similar situation.

Long-Term Planning

Caregivers need to be included in planning long-term care goals, because their lives are affected by the patient's plan of care. Discussions need to include the spectrum of options that are available, from acquiring more care in the home to the possible need for placement in a long-term care facility. Frequently, caregivers are reluctant to express their own concerns or needs and place priority on the patient. However, the inability to plan one's own life can place an undue amount of stress on the caregiver. (See Chapter 7 for the Caregiver's Bill of Rights.)

Some Personal Accounts of Health Team Members

The following statements by a community health nurse, a nutritionist, a hospice volunteer and a social worker reflect a few of the experiences and feelings that any home health caregiver may have at one time or another. They emphasize positive and negative aspects of home health care. A most grisly example of home health care stories, in which a visiting nurse is shot to death, appears in Chapter 9, which centers on safety and liability issues. Though caregivers may not always be risking their lives to provide home care, they do frequently encounter many a surprise at the doorsteps of private dwellings.

Hugs or havoc

For the past four years, I have been a community health nurse. This area of nursing has been both rewarding and an eye-opening experience. Many factors affect your patient and the care you give. Working in the hospital setting, you enjoy a controlled environment. You can go to work, do your job and, for the most part, afterward focus on your own life. In community health, you think of almost every patient continuously. You are part of their family to an extent. But mostly the conflict you deal with daily is money. Finances greatly affect your patient care. Program budgets and funding affecting home health aide time is a constant worry, as well as denial from private insurance sources for something that would benefit your patient. You need to consider a person's supply of wound-care dressings, food, diapers, formula, even utilities. In the hospital your patients are fed, clothed, clean and warm. You could go to the supply closet and grab anything you need.

Never in a million years did I imagine myself going to insect-infested homes, or cluttered and dirty homes, but I do, to do my job. You begin to realize that these are the patients' homes, their castle. It is what they are used to, without posing a health risk. When new nurses start with our agency, I make it a point to take them to these types of homes. I emphasize to the nurses that this is their patients' turf, not ours, unlike in the hospital, where they conform to our terms. Now we as the guests in their homes must conform to their terms. We need to respect their homes, no matter what.

The thrill of being a visiting nurse is that you never know what to expect. Your days are totally unpredictable. Some days your visits are quiet and routine. These days you appreciate giving and getting that well-deserved hug, or spending extra time talking to a patient who is lonely, or spending that needed time for patient-teaching. But then there are the days of havoc. Every visit is draining and demanding of your nursing ability.

You either love or hate community health nursing. I love it. You cannot get into this job and think it will be a stable, constant day. You learn to be flexible and creative very quickly.

---*Teresa Vaccaro, RN*

What's cooking

When I was doing a lot of home care in nutrition, I encountered some tricky situations. For example, I was working with a poor, inner-city woman on a nutrition plan. She had several health problems that needed to be addressed through an improved diet, so I sat with her for hours, planning the most inexpensive purchases of good foods and explaining what to prepare and why this was important. The woman was nice, totally receptive. At the end of all our discussions, I asked her: "Well, do you think you really can make these meals on the $20 a week as we figured out?" And the woman said, "Sure, but not this month." I was puzzled. "What do you mean, not this month?" "Oh," she replied, "because this month I couldn't pay my gas bill, so I can't cook."

---Name withheld

You have to be there

Each day as I set up my schedule of home visits, I know that my work fills a very special need in the community—one that cannot be filled in any other way. To sit in a client's kitchen, perhaps over a cup of tea, sharing knowledge of community resources with a disabled person who may have no access to the complicated world of social services, is satisfying and has immediate impact in that home. For the homebound or chronically ill, this informal, nonthreatening way of helping creates bonds of friendship and trust. Whether my job requires obtaining respite care for the overwhelmed mother of a severely disabled child, or getting assistance to a wheelchair-bound person with MS, considering alternatives to nursing-home placement—well, you just have to be there to see how rewarding that can be for a home care professional.

--- Joan Powers, MSW, LCSW

Chapter 5

No job too odd or too small

   Human beings enter this world at the beginning of their lives and exit at the end. What occurs between those two mileposts is a journey. Most often, people join their lives and their energies in order to make the journey meaningful and to insure companionship through both the easy and difficult terrain. However, there is one point in each of our journeys through which we must pass unaccompanied: the final step that marks the separation of beings. The process of preparing for that time can be stressful for the person leaving and the persons remaining behind. The time spent completing this process is often accompanied by fear and pain and is likely to be the most intimate and private moments of one's life.
It is natural, then, that I have chosen to support others during this process, as I have always felt that my role in life is to be one who makes the journey easier in any way possible for those in physical and/or emotional pain. I feel my role as a hospice volunteer is that of providing an unconditionally supportive connection with persons in the process of severing their connections with this world and each other.
   Preconceived notions about how to provide that support while truly respecting the individual must be thrown out the window. In order to insure that the connection provided is supportive and unqualified, the hospice volunteer must open his or her heart and mind to comprehend spoken and unspoken needs of the dying person and the person's family. As a hospice companion, I have been called upon to perform a variety of roles. For one woman, I was companion and manicurist. We spent many hours sitting in her backyard comparing recipes, housekeeping hints and polishing nails. We also took one final car ride to various farm and flower markets in the area, as she enjoyed beautiful things. I was her confidante and sounding board when she experienced anger and frustration at becoming physically less capable of mobility and strength.
   No matter what role I undertook, I remained first and foremost my most open and honest self, which has put me face to face with a multitude of positive and negative emotions.

---Cary Katz, MA

86

Home Care: An Ad-lib Performance

As a physical therapist (PT) since 1982, I have been fortunate to participate in the many facets of my profession. Hospital-based care, private practice, outpatient care and home care have afforded wonderful opportunities for great interactions at many different levels. This is reflected in the facilitation of the well-being of people in the healing process.

As an academician, I have been charged to foster the development of future PTs. What an incredible responsibility this is amidst the changing health-care dynamics! Versatility and an insatiable quest for lifelong learning are the themes of my teaching. The acquisition of rehabilitation skills is only a small step in the process. The inquiry "beyond technique" allows for PT/client interaction in a way that only time can bring about. The foundation is where my role as a teacher is underscored, yet through this, an infusion of the human condition is of utmost importance.

Home care is where the heart of the matter is viewed. There is a certain humbleness that takes place when you enter the home of another. The expertise behind the health care practitioner is the key to the entrance, yet the ability to make a powerful contribution to the individuals in the household takes place in multifaceted ways. A certain examination of one's biases or judgments toward living conditions is imperative. Does the way we treat the client have an impact, because of certain living styles? How are we affected by the demands of the family?

Today, clients are discharged from the hospital at an accelerated pace and what we witness is an *acute* situation that prevails in the home. The disruption in daily family routines and the focus on the client are all parts of the process that we see as we render care. The amount of equipment necessary to manage the client is certainly not similar to buying new furniture. The content of the family household attempts to remain the same amidst the architectural changes.

The family requires a voice as the client is treated. This voice needs to be encouraged and the permission to experience the many facets of change explored. All in all, home care really is a "family affair." An analogy that I like to use is a performance. A dance, when choreographed, may need to be changed before the opening of the first act. Intermission may require additional alterations based on the "players." The orchestration of events may present with many new openings that make the dance more exciting, depressing, or overwhelming for the actors. Yet the piece is performed and the audience receives it. Interpretation of the dance may take many different shapes.

It is in this "receiving" that we, as health care professionals, facilitate in the "orchestration" of events. We can be catalysts in the design of the dance. How we script the dance may take us into unchartered territory. Are we able to accept the journey? Are we free to travel the roads that are unpaved? Therein lie many discoveries that provide us with both personal and professional growth from home care.

----*Mary Lou Galantino, MS, PT*

In conclusion, we regret that space is too limited to offer hundreds of personal stories of health care team members, and that very often professional and assistive roles are described more perfunctorily than they may actually be. That is, of course, because human beings interact and relate to each other on so many levels, which makes cut-and-dried roles impossible. Throw in tremendous knowledge, caring, empathy, and accountability, and you quadruplicate all the layers of interaction that already exist. Unless you live on a cragged ledge in the Himalayas, the title of this chapter stands: *Never the "Lone Ranger."*

Summary

- The patient is the most important team member.

- Patients' significant others become part of the treatment and may affect the course of treatment positively or negatively.

- In the home, the role of both the patient and significant others is generally more concrete than in institutional settings.

- The interdisciplinary treatment team is a group of various professionals whose collective goal is to help improve the patient's condition.

- The nurse is responsible for monitoring the patient's medical condition, educating the patient in regard to his or her care, and making recommendations and referrals to other disciplines, pending the physician's approval.

- The medical social worker assists the patient and family with psychosocial counseling to facilitate coping with illness or disability. The social worker also gives the patient and family information about community resources that may be beneficial to the patient.

- The physical therapist assesses the degree to which a patient has been physically debilitated by illness and prescribes and performs a course of physical therapy.

- The occupational therapist employs corrective devices and other equipment to help the patient regain functioning in daily living skills and activities.

- The respiratory therapist works with patients with breathing problems by teaching them to perform appropriate exercises using respiratory devices, such as incentive spirometer.

- The IV therapist is trained in the use and monitoring of intravenous therapies; increasingly these therapies are used by patients at home.

- The physician directs medical care of the patient.

- The dietitian prescribes diets and helps patients adapt new dietary needs to their particular lifestyle.

- Team members need to educate patients and communicate with other team members regarding their areas of expertise and professional capabilities.

- An interdisciplinary health care team is a group of individuals representing different professions who work in complementary capacities to facilitate the total wellness of the patient.

- None of us are lone practitioners; we are all members of a larger effort.

- Parochialism, inevitably, works to the detriment of the patient.

- Becoming knowledgeable about other disciplines will enhance your own professional growth and improve patient care.

- Be clear as to how you see your professional role.

- Know how your agency defines your role.

- We are each ambassadors for our respective professions.

- Leaders need to spell out roles and responsibilities of team members.

- Organizations need to develop clear job descriptions to help eliminate confusion and boundary disputes.

- Many organizations have only rudimentary vehicles encouraging team members to interact, eg, referrals and access to documentation. Make yourself available for consultation with other team members.

- The best antidote to territoriality is the development of positive interdisciplinary relations.

- Be aware of an organization's cultural values and its historical treatment of various disciplines.

Chapter 6

The Home Health Aide and Ancillary Services

A certain man went down from Jerusalem to Jericho, and fell among thieves, which stripped him of his raiment and wounded him, and departed, leaving him half dead. And by chance there came down a certain priest that way...and passed by on the other side. And likewise a Levite.... But a certain Samaritan...went to him, and bound up his wounds...and took care of him.
Luke 10: 30-33

Pat and Joe Hunter were an average suburban couple in their early sixties. After working for nearly 40 years for a large corporation and raising four children, Joe decided to take an early retirement. Joe and Pat brought a mobile home and planned to tour the Pacific Northwest. Because Joe's job entailed much traveling, there had been little time for vacations. A month after retiring, Joe was diagnosed with pancreatic cancer. Not only did Joe face a limited prognosis and the loss of an opportunity that he and Pat had worked years to earn, neither Joe nor Pat had ever been seriously ill and had no idea how to cope with a terminal illness. Realizing that there was little to be done, Joe's physician made a referral to hospice.

Following the nurse's initial visit and assessment, the first member of the hospice to visit was Teresa W., an experienced home health aide who exuded confidence and warmth. Although Joe and Pat had never been in this situation, Teresa had been there with families countless times. Teresa was able to show Joe and Pat that it was manageable and gave them confidence in their own abilities. Joe and Pat began to experience a level of comfort that they had not had since before Joe was diagnosed. No longer were they at the mercy of treatment schedules or side effects.

Suddenly, they were able to pursue their old interests with the only intervening factor being Joe's feeling up to whatever it was. Joe had a couple of good months. During that time, they were able to visit Joe's sister in Florida, see several Broadway shows, and have plenty of time for Joe to play poker with his pals. It was a large and welcome infusion of normalcy. Along with other hospice team members, Teresa was instrumental in showing Joe and Pat that they were, indeed, capable of enjoying Joe's final days with grace and dignity.

Teresa worked with the nurse to assist Pat and Joe in making this important transition. She was able to make Joe more comfortable with his need for physical care, and she was able to teach Pat many aspects of patient care. Teresa's presence for a few hours, several times a week, was an enormous help to Pat, and enabled Pat to get out to run errands, see friends or just take a rest. During the several months of Joe's illness, Teresa became almost like a trusted friend or family member. As Joe's condition continued to deteriorate, hospice care was instrumental in keeping Joe at home. Staying at home was extremely important to both Joe and Pat. When Joe died, Pat wrote to hospice thanking everyone for the assistance which she and Joe had received. Pat wrote that without the physical help and emotional support which Teresa had given, she could not have managed to keep Joe at home. Teresa had helped to give Joe his last wish.

The home health aide may be considered the cornerstone — the "Mom," if you will — of the treatment team. Although this is not to slight in any way the role of the physician, nurse, or other caregivers, it is difficult to overestimate the importance of the care provided by home health aides when many patients will return home unable to care for their own physical needs. Said Ann Healy of the VNA of Central New Jersey, "The home health aide is often the first person that the family or patient asks for."

The aide provides the personal and physical care services that form the foundation of the patient's wellness, and is responsible for performing for the patient activities of daily living, such as bathing, eating, or dressing. The certified home health aide (CHHA) completes a course of study and generally works for an agency under the direction of a registered nurse. Requirements for certification are generally 60 to 75 hours of course work, but requirements vary from state to state. Although the training time is limited, the course is intensive and the material covered almost global in nature. A sampling of the subject areas taught include the measurement of vital signs; personal care, which includes oral hygiene, dressing, bathing, feeding, perineal care, shaving; infection control; appropriate handling of medical waste and the implementation of sterile technique; proper reporting of the patient's condition; and familiarity with medical equipment. In addition, the home health aide may perform light housekeeping duties, such as personal laundry, food shopping, dishwashing, dusting, and vacuuming. In general, these services must be for the patient and not other family members.

Although the role the home health aide plays in the total treatment scheme is invaluable, unfortunately the value society assigns to this role often falls far short of its true worth. The home health aide profession has been characterized by relatively low pay rates, high turnover rates, and low rates of job satisfaction.

In 1989, John F. Kennedy Jr., Esq., founded *Reaching Up*, an organization dedicated to upgrading the status and recognition given to persons providing direct care services to the disabled. *Reaching Up* states that its mission is to support the education and career advancement of direct care workers who provide health, education and social services to individuals with disabilities. *Reaching Up* is composed of three major components:

- **The Kennedy Fellows Program**: provides scholarships and mentoring to direct care workers enrolled at CUNY (City University of New York) and SUNY (State University of New York) colleges. Each year 100 Kennedy Fellows are selected.
- **The Consortium for the Study of Disabilities**: provides small grants to colleges to develop training programs in rehabilitation services. More than 1,000 worker/students are enrolled in more than 50 new courses and sponsored academic programs each year.
- **The Center for Workforce Development**: provides technical assistance to human service agencies to help develop comprehensive workforce plans and improve relationships between their consumers and direct care staff.

A goal of the organization is to increase the level of professionalism and respect accorded to those involved in direct care. *Reaching Up* believes that creating an improvement in status and working conditions for direct care workers will affect a concomitant improvement in the quality of services received by the consumer. *Reaching Up* recognizes that direct care workers in the health care field do not face a "glass ceiling"; they face a real wall. The efforts of *Reaching Up* are making a significant contribution toward the creation of a career ladder for those in this field. The presence of an organization such as this in health care is long overdue.

As with the other disciplines, the home health aide's role is determined by the patient's plan of care, and services will vary with the patient's condition and special needs. When a person is debilitated, either through hospitalization or chronic illness, often the availability of home health services will determine whether or not a person is able to return home. The ultimate success or failure of the patient's treatment is inextricably bound to the quality of care the home health aide provides.

The Homemaker

The important distinction between a home health aide and a homemaker is that home health aides are primarily responsible for patients' personal care, feeding, dressing, etc., whereas the homemaker maintains the physical environment, eg, dusting, cooking, shopping. The home health aide may perform some of these tasks, but they are more limited and directly related to patient care. Most insurance companies and third-party payers require personal care as a condition for reimbursement. Many patients need education regarding the differences between home health aides and homemakers and are confused regarding the distinction between the two. Patients are often hard-pressed to understand why the home health aide does not polish the family heirlooms and why the homemaker cannot give a bath.

Both the tasks the home health aide and the homemaker perform are akin to tasks mothers perform in traditional families. Although the role of mothers in society is assigned a high emotional value, there is little corresponding economic value placed upon the contribution of their work. Several years ago, I met a young woman who was a Fulbright scholar, and who, at the time, was staying home caring for her two small daughters. Maria said, "Many people ask me, Why are you not pursuing your career? Why are you staying home with children? I must ask them, What could be more important than the care of my children?" In home care, we might ask what could be more important than ensuring the physical care and comfort of our patients.

The Hierarchy of Home Health Care

When Maslow gave us his theory of a hierarchy of human needs, he also gave us a blueprint that works beautifully in relation to the priority of health care needs. Maslow's theory proposes that human beings must first attend to their physiological needs such as hunger, thirst, sleep, shelter, etc., before they can pursue more abstract needs such as mastery, belongingness, and self-actualization. Nowhere more than in health care do we see Maslow's theory validated. As we deal with people whose physical capabilities and capacity to care for themselves are compromised, we realize that until the patient is fed, changed, and dressed, any attempts at remediation are doomed to failure. Once we have constructed this foundation of care, we can move on to the remediation of illness, physical rehabilitation, long-term planning, attention to family and psychosocial issues, and spiritual needs. The home health aide, together with the patient, family, and friends, will form this infrastructure of care.

The Home Health Aide as an Emotional Support to the Patient

As the health care system continues to tighten its belt and lengths of stay continue their downward spiral, greater numbers of patients will return home needing as much or more assistance than they needed in the hospital. For many patients and family members, this is a frightening prospect indeed. Many patients will be returning home to significant others or family caregivers who are elderly and frail themselves. At other times it may be that a young, inexperienced mother is bringing her first child home, often after less than 24 hours in the hospital. In the world of dual working parents, the "sandwich generation," and families separated by long distances, some will return to situations where family and significant others will be limited in the amount of assistance they can give. In some instances, there is no caregiver at all. In most instances, the person returning home will be changed somehow from the person that the caregiver knew. The patient and family confront issues of dependency and helplessness and must find ways of coping. For patient and family, the transition from the hospital to home can be a frightening and disconcerting time.

On one level, the patient and family will be challenged to find the physical resources to deal with the patient's altered condition. On an emotional level, the challenge is to deal with the pain, sense of loss, and frustration, and the many small "deaths" associated with chronic or terminal illness. As illness and natural aging progress, the patient and family must deal with altered physical presence and a decreased functioning ability. All of these changes create stress for the patient and his support system. In essence, the treatment team will meet the patient and family at a time of crisis, or at the very least, disruption. Here the home health aide, along with other team members, will go beyond meeting the physiological and treatment needs of the patient and become a source of emotional support for the patient and the family.

At 83, Charlie Morgan had been known to the local VNA for the past ten years. He and his wife, Sally, lived in a senior citizen apartment complex. Both Sally and Charlie had multiple physical problems, and had been hospitalized for extensive periods. Charlie's problems were primarily cardiac, whereas Sally had had several strokes. Following these hospitalizations, the couple had been seen by the visiting nurse for a short period, usually 3 weeks.

These short encounters were to create lasting impressions. The nurse, home health aide, and physical therapist were to fall under Charlie and Sally's spell.

Charlie and Sally had that "caring for the caregiver touch" that so many of us in the helping professions find irresistible. In short, they both loved people, and something like chronic illness was not about to prevent them from doing what they had done all their lives: care for others. They knew whose husband had the flu, who had a bad back, who was scheduled for promotion, and, what's more, they really cared. The staff at the VNA was ready to consider adoption proceedings.

When Sally died, the social worker from the VNA helped Charlie get on one of the long-term Medicaid community care plans designed to assist nursing home-eligible persons in their own homes. In a beautifully designed program that provides many of the services available in long-term care facilities such as nursing visits, physical therapy, social work, and home health aide, Charlie thrived.

Charlie got off to a rough start on the program when they assigned 21-year-old Kelly to be his home health aide. Charlie was embarrassed at the prospect of having someone so young care for him, but didn't want to say so. Charlie was taken off guard when Kelly quickly helped him put his life back together. Suddenly, his wash was done, his apartment straightened, and his meals cooked. Once again there was a pleasant, caring person in his life.

Kelly found that she had come to look forward to the days when she would see Charlie. Kelly's "inner child" never tired of hearing the stories of Little Charlie's birth 50 years before when the doctor had stayed all night, drinking gallons of coffee and playing "My Wild Irish Rose" on Sally's old spinet, of how they had lost a home in the depths of the Depression, but had always managed to keep the spinet, of hearing the history of all Charlie and Sally's possessions from Sally's cranberry glass collection to all the orphan furniture they found and resurrected. Some-where in the process, Kelly and Charlie knew they were retracing the fabric of a life.

As time passed, Charlie grew increasingly dependent upon his nitroglycerin capsules, seemed quieter, and even spoke less of Sally. Kelly was with Charlie when he had a massive coronary and died. They had been together for 2 years, and during that time Kelly had done much more for Charlie than simply his laundry and personal care. She had helped him to achieve an important personal goal: to remain in his own home and determine his own way of life.

Although it is relatively easy to calculate the cost benefit of maintaining someone like Charlie Morgan at home as opposed the cost involved in a long-term care facility, it is far more challenging, albeit not impossible, to factor in the differences in a patient's quality of life remaining at home can achieve. The desire to remain in one's home is almost universal. If there are few atheists on the battlefield, there is an equally small number of patients who wish to relinquish their homes in favor of the nursing home. This is not to say that long-term care facilities and nursing homes have not moved light years in the past decade in their abilities to provide highly specialized care or approximate a homelike environment; nor that in many instances, it is the setting that will be best able to meet certain patient's care needs. Yet, the desire to remain in one's home is one that is dear to many patients' hearts.

An Interview with a Home Health Aide

Anita P., 25, has been a certified home health aide for four years. She had been attending nursing school, took a leave of absence, and plans to return. Her work as an HHA, she said, will definitely help her in her future nursing career.

Q: *What types of patients do you have now?*
A: I have two assignments, one an 11-year-old boy with a seizure disorder, and a 19-year-old boy with muscular dystrophy.

Q: *What do you do for them?*
A: The younger boy needs help walking up and down stairs, etc. I prepare his dinner and make sure he doesn't hurt himself if he has a seizure. I only give him medications if his mother measures them out first, and if he has a wound, I'm not to clean or change his bandages. My job may be characterized as a "precautionary" measure. I've been with the older boy for 3 years now, and I'm used to his pattern. He cannot move a muscle except for his head, so he needs me to help him bathe, shampoo his hair, clean his teeth, and use the bedpan. I cook for him and feed him, too. I'm there 4 hours a day.

Q: *How did you first react to these patients when you started your assignments?*
A: I never really expected them to be at home. In the hospital, but not home. I feel nervous at first, but generally I like to work in the patients' homes. But I remember having to fill in for another home health aide to take care of an elderly woman who needed all kinds of assistance. The whole house smelled of urine, and when I first saw this woman, she was covered in urine. The house was full of boxes and clutter, and there was barely any room to move. It wasn't a pleasant experience.

Q: *What is another example of something that surprised you on the job?*
A: Sometimes the reaction of family members to the patient. One hospice patient with Alzheimer's lived with her son who did nothing for her. One day he said to me, "Don't come; I have jury duty." I asked when he was going to feed his mother the day of his jury duty, and he said he just wouldn't feed her until that night! He was nice to me, but it was really weird.

Q: *That sounds like a referral to the social worker. How do you get along with the nurses and social workers and other team members?*
A: I look at them very highly. What they do is tough, just like what I do is tough. You need a good working relationship with them. It takes a lot of communication. You have to keep them posted on what has been happening and your fear of what might happen, such as with hospice patients. It's rare for me to actually see the social workers. I find I deal mainly with the nurses and physical therapists.

Q: *What is one of the limitations of your job?*
A: Many patients don't understand that you can't drive them places in your car, only the family's car and only in an emergency. They'll say to you, "I won't tell if you won't." You have to be very assertive.

Q: *What other quality does a home health aide need to be successful?*
A: Compassion. No one can teach you that. You have to put yourself in the patient's situation and physically learn what is most comfortable for you and the patient. You set up the routine — what is easiest, most efficient for the two of you. That all comes with time.

Other Members of the Health Care Team

In addition to the homemakers and home health aides, agencies send out nurse's aides, physical and occupational therapy assistants, "chore persons," massage therapists, companions, and volunteers.

Organizations, agencies, and registries may differ significantly on the tasks assigned to each assistant. For example, some nurse's aides are not allowed to pour and administer medications to patients, whereas others must do this because they are the only caregivers on duty at the times a patient receives medications. Directions for the nurse's aide may be cooperatively decided upon by the nurse and the patient's family in order to reduce any liabilities (see Chapter 9).

One of the major difficulties inherent in the work of the ancillary or assistive care provider is a "stepping on toes" situation. Unlicensed assistive personnel (UAPs) brought about much controversy among the professionals. Although home health aides and homemakers are usually well-regarded and valued, and nurses have always worked with nurse's aides who perform many of the mundane duties (bedmaking, etc.) that free the nurse to do professional tasks, the emergence of PTAs, OTAs and other assistants have raised some important questions.

Given that the health care team's goal is to help improve the client's condition, nurses tend to object to "technical assistants" who are minimally trained to do nursing tasks and who work for less money, thus creating a thorny competition. When a medical facility turns nursing work over to "techs," nurses believe the patients are at risk. One registered nurse explained her feeling toward aides and technicians in a letter to the editors of the Asbury Park Press (April 29, 1995):

> "In an attempt to save money, registered nurses are being replaced by aides and 'technicians,' especially in the critical care units. This means that you, the patient, are now being taken care of in a more critical area by less-trained personnel. The hospitals feel they need to employ fewer nurses because these 'techs' can do the 'busy' work that nurses do, such as give baths and change linen.
> Do you, the consumer, realize that when I'm bathing you, I'm reassessing your condition and observing minute changes...listening to your lungs, rubbing your back, and discussing your condition, teaching, or listening to what you have to say to me, the registered nurse. These 'techs' are also responsible for watching heart monitors, which detect life-threatening changes in your heart's rhythm.
> I'm also your patient advocate, making sure your needs and concerns are being addressed to the physician and coordinating your care with my assessments. I'm there to mediate and at times 'interpret' what your physician tells you."

Much of the same sentiment on assistants applies to the home care nurse, physical and occupational therapist, and other professionals. One possibility is to allow the assistants to work under the direct supervision and in the presence of the professional, which, of course, defeats an agency's or facility's desire to cut expenses and staff. Another is to permit working assistants in the case of persons in a professional training program. The controversy has just begun, and solutions have not yet been reached. What becomes policy in the hospitals, however, may well filter into home care.

This is a legitimate cause for concern, especially in light of the fact that home caregivers do not necessarily have the immediate support and consulting potential that hospital personnel enjoy. The nurse's aide or home health aide on a night shift alone with an incapacitated patient may not be able to reach anyone except emergency room staff or the first-aid squad team, neither of which is appropriate for anything but true emergencies. Home care, then, may become as critical as the care given in the intensive care unit of a hospital. The home health team needs to pull together at all times — and make the home a supportive central station that helps clients heal.

Massage Therapy

Usually licensed in most states, the massage therapy practitioner or certified massage therapist (CMT) may be called upon to make a home visit. Now being recommended by physicians and other caregivers, massage releases chronic tension and pain, eases muscle tightness, reduces inflammation, and in some cases limits the formation of scar tissue, improves the circulation, increases flexibility of the joints, and reduces physical and mental fatigue. In addition, as a technique of positive touch, massage relieves stress and symptoms aggravated by anxiety and insomnia.

As in any alternative care technique, massage therapists are ethically required to avoid false claims on the benefits of massage and acknowledge their professional limitations, referring a client to an appropriate medical professional when necessary. And as in any caregiving profession, massage therapists are to conduct themselves professionally and appropriately at all times, and they are expected to cooperate with all health professionals. In addition to its Code of Ethics, the Association of Bodywork and Massage Professionals (ABMP) expects its members to keep accurate records and carry liability insurance.

Summary

- Recognize the importance of the services you provide. Often these services are the deciding factor in whether a patient can be maintained at home.
- The amount of time you spend with patients may be greater than that of any other team member. You may be aware of circumstances or problems no other team member knows.
- Be clear as to your responsibilities and duties.
- Learn to trust your own instincts. If you feel something is wrong, it may well be.
- Help educate patients and families. Remember, they may not understand your role.
- Make self-care a priority. You can care for no one until you care for yourself.
- Perform your duties with complete professionalism. Your work forms the basis on which all other services depend.
- Work on your own professional development. An excellent home health aide is one of the most sought-after team members.
- Develop a support system to suit your own needs. It could be other home health aides, family or friends.
- Find a mentor. Be sure it is someone you admire and respect. Learn from him or her.
- Communicate with other team members. It works to the benefit of the patient and the team.

Chapter 7

Care for the Caregiver: The Joys and Problems of Doing Good

If I can stop one heart from breaking,
I shall not live in vain;
If I can ease one life the aching,
Or cool one pain,
Or help one fainting robin
Unto his nest again,
I shall not live in vain.
Emily Dickinson

Caregiving ranks as a service of premium value among human beings. Self-care is an obligation in honor of caregiving. It is logical and universally correct to realize that as patients need physical and psychological attention, so do caregivers need to receive some kind of nurturance for themselves that goes beyond the patient's progress and restoration to health. Mary Catherine Bateson, author of *Composing a Life*, points out in her book that it is "not easy to learn to cherish oneself when one's life has been organized around cherishing others or when all the cherishing has been delegated to someone else." But, she continues, "a little cherishing of the self is translated into responsible behavior, even a way of caring for others..."

Many of us were taught relentlessly, including as a rule of fifth-grade English grammar, to put ourselves last. We were taught to say, "My friends and I," not "I and my friends." Impressed by the idea that to put oneself ahead of others is selfish, individuals who choose the helping professions as adults all too frequently believe they must defer to the needs of their patients at all costs. This they believe and revere as dedication.

In *The Healing Power of Doing Good*, by Allan Luks and Peggy Payne, physician David Sobel and psychologist Robert Ornstein are quoted as saying, "The greatest surprise of human evolution may be that

the highest form of selfishness is selflessness." Dedication that depletes
the caregiver to the point of illness or non-function turns into foolishness
and wastefulness. To be selfless to that degree implies that the caregiver
has misinterpreted the fundamental command to "Love thy neighbor as
thyself."

Luks, whose background includes the Peace Corps, the Institute for
the Advancement of Health, and Big Brothers/Big Sisters of New York
City, describes a "helper's high" as a result of caring briefly or at length
for others, perhaps the finest way to care for ourselves. The "helper's
high," a feeling akin to euphoria, high self-esteem and profound
gratification, has been touted as therapeutic for the caregiver and a
reason for persisting in a health profession despite potentially
traumatizing and exhausting aspects. The most successful caregiver is
one who feels good about his or her working life and knows how to
sustain it and thrive because of it.

A healthy brand of "selfishness" involves self-care that follows
Maslow's hierarchy of needs as well as a simple teaching of Judaism,
Christianity, Islam and other faiths: because our bodies are "temples,"
our souls part of a universal divinity, and we are to treat others as we
want to be treated ourselves, we must first keep ourselves going. To
prepare well for an emergency or stressful situation, remember that
airline flight attendants instruct adult passengers to put on their own
oxygen masks first, then put the masks on children or others who need
help.

Caregivers often think that caring in itself can infuse some kind of
bionic ability in the face of illness or other adversity. The famous
declaration of a little boy carrying another boy on his back — "He ain't
heavy, he's my brother" (attributed to the legend of Father Flanagan's
"Boys Town") — offers inspiration and the knowledge that when the
caring is intense enough, the actual labor of the caregiver seems to
diminish. What we tend not to allow for, however, is the reality that
dictates that one cannot "carry" another indefinitely, because one will
require refreshment for himself sooner or later in order *to continue the
care of the other.* In his poem "Vigil Strange I Kept on the Field One
Night," Walt Whitman reminds us to praise ourselves for our work and
then give it over to a Higher Power: "I faithfully loved you and cared for
you living. I think we shall surely meet again." In addition to self-
crediting, Stuart Wilde gets to the practical core of things in his book,
The Trick to Money is Having Some!, Wilde writes, "You learned to love
others, but in so doing allowed the world to walk all over you....In
loving others you forgot to love yourself....What a drag."

Part of the refreshment for caregivers involves managing the intensity
of the work day after day. In a chapter of *Oncology Social Work: A
Clinician's Guide,* one of the authors, Naomi M. Stearns, MSW, writes

on this professional issue for social workers, but the concepts are applicable to any health professional, especially those in home care where work intensity can be every bit the high drama of an inner-city emergency room.

> "Oncology social workers frequently are asked to explain how they manage the intensity of their work or time. This query is generally followed by observations that the oncology social worker must either qualify for sainthood or find the work inordinately depressing. This is not a description that most social workers find useful, especially when new to the field of oncology. However, these well-intentioned components do force staff to consider both the positive and negative impacts of the work. Identifying sources of stress and developing strategies to manage the physical and emotional aspects of the work are crucial to maintaining professional and personal balance."

Balance first demands understanding that, in becoming caregivers, professionals wish to do their best, but not at the expense of trying to achieve the impossible with a patient or putting themselves in prolonged physical or emotional danger. Balance, in fact, mandates self-care and protection, for the problems may creep up and accumulate slowly or they may hit like a storm. Some of the issues include an unrealistic amount of care required to be given by one person; lack of support and/or resources; a frail or at-risk caregiver; job isolation or "homeboundedness"; lack of respite service; interference of significant others; environmental deficits; patient abuse; caregiver abuse; patient/caregiver conflict; difficulties with work requirements (shift hours, etc.), and lack of agency or registry support. It is worth considering that these difficulties may arise either from reality shock or burnout.

Reality Shock

Author Marlene Kramer identified and described what she called "reality shock": a reaction particularly of new health-care graduates who, upon entry into the workforce, suddenly have to cope with situations for which they feel they were not prepared in school. Because new graduates tend to concentrate on skill and routine mastery of professional concepts as they were taught, they may be morally outraged at what goes on in "real" practice, feel betrayed by teachers and employers, and require a new socialization in their field so they do not alienate their peers or others, or create conflict for themselves.

Internships and in-depth orientation programs often provide crucial initiation into a particular workplace or professional circumstance. Preparation for home care, however, may be an impossible dream because no instructor or program leader has every possible type of encounter nailed down for observation. Unlike Henry Kissinger, who once said, "There can't be a crisis next week — my schedule for next week is full," health caregivers live constantly at the whim and mercy of crises, or at very least, the unexpected. The best way to prepare for whatever life in the field serves up is to have an arsenal of memories of other peoples' experiences, knowledge of what to do in an emergency or difficult situations, and critically thought-out plans for action ahead of time. Add strong self-care skills and compassion, and most of the battle is already won.

Burnout

The term "burnout" was first used in 1973 by Dr. Herbert Freudenberger, author of *Burn Out: The High Cost of Achievement*, to describe a state of exhaustion brought about by working too intensely without regard to one's own needs. Although any profession may be subject to burnout, the helping professions are especially at risk for this syndrome. In the course of a week, the average health professional will see more suffering and illness than most people will see in a lifetime. This would appear to be a recipe for disaster.

Freudenberger wrote in 1980, "The work of the helping professions is taxing and tough. The helper has come to his profession with visions of a supportive institution peopled with wise superiors, and cooperative patients, students or clients. What he finds instead is red tape, harried administrators, intractable cases. No one has prepared him for this. No one comes forward to ameliorate his feelings of inadequacy."

The issue of burnout becomes even more problematic as the tightening of the health-care dollar, the chronicity of the problems encountered, and a myriad of psychosocial problems make the home health worker's job increasingly difficult. Emotional stressors facing the home caregiver are not usually present in other areas of health care. The hospital or outpatient clinic worker does not ordinarily have first-hand knowledge of a client's living situation, and consequently, does not have to deal with it. But the home health nurse or other caregiver, who encounters a patient suffering from abuse or neglect or who is simply unable to care for himself, makes it her business to mobilize all resources to help that patient.

Whereas the nurse, social worker, therapist, and other home caregivers take pride in their ability to make significant improvements in the lives of people with staggering, multiple needs, it is often these (as well as lay caregivers) — the ones with the highest standards for themselves and others — who are most prone to burnout.

One writer and former nun, Mary L. Brasseur, recounted her experience caring for her senile father-in-law, who lived with her for 2 years before he died of cancer. It is not unlike the stories many nurses and therapists tell when they stood on the brink of near-senselessness resulting from good motivation and lack of the healthy brand of selfishness.

> "I do my best to see to his comfort and happiness, but he insists on making himself the total focus of my life and this drives me crazy....Was I so smug in thinking I was kind, patient and could handle anything?...I have come to the point where I can only abide him....I should not be making commitments for which I am physically and emotionally unfit and because I wallow in guilt, I find it hard to go back on them....What was it you said, Lord, It is easy to love the lovable; what merit is there in that?...So here I am full of contention and complaints and contrition...polishing my patience, exhuming my endurance and searching for my lost serenity...."

Furthermore, caregiving tasks that demand the strength of an ox and the cunning David needed to slay Goliath may be only half the picture. Burnout, or the final stage of stress run amok, has been attributable to the dysfunctional workplace — a kind of "poisoned well."

Little in a caregiver's education prepares him or her for surviving in organizations that let pathological work environments fester. Most caregivers enter their fields with a *joie de vivre* that may quickly be shot down by any number of organizational dysfunctions: work overload, non-cooperation, professional jealousy, harassment, boundary violations, poor or "control-mentality" managers, intense and inappropriate competition, fears ranging from malpractice to losing one's job in a downsizing maneuver, etc. In the sense of Eldridge Cleaver's words, "If you are not part of the solution, you are part of the problem," the culture of an organization that does not empower the well-motivated, well-trained workers empowers the "monsters."

Maladaptive behaviors ensue. The workplace comes to reflect the dysfunction that has infiltrated the American family unit. Consider the dilemma of the caregiver who works for an agency that allows "monsters" to thrive undaunted and then arrives at a client's home to discover more dysfunction. Because the caregiver has no control over the agency or the client's domain, he or she is now flirting dangerously with stress that may lead to burnout.

One of the greatest resources for counteracting burnout is a strong network of social, familial, fraternal and professional supports. Supportive relationships provide a vehicle for dealing with stress. They offer advice based on empathetic understanding, and they help establish a less emotional, more realistic appraisal of one's own efforts and predicaments.

The support systems, then, create pathways leading away from some of the isolation and reality shock one may experience while still in training. In many ways, today's professional finds himself at a disadvantage when compared with the master craftsman of the Middle Ages. Author Constance Brittain Bouchard wrote in her book, *Antiquity and the Middle Ages*, that the guilds to which the craftsman belonged fashioned an educational system, standards of excellence, conferred status, and a sense of community among members. As members progressed through the stages of apprentice, journeyman, and master craftsman, they received the instruction and guidance of the established masters. Although our educational system mirrors the guild system in the way it confers degrees, the process usually terminates as soon as the degree is conferred. In short, we often lack mentors.

Mentoring: A Good Mentor Is Hard To Find

Our present-day concept of mentoring comes from the story of Odysseus in Greek mythology. In this tale, Odysseus entrusts the care of his son Telemachus to his friend and advisor, Mentor, while he journeys far from home. For Mentor, the care of Telemachus is a sacred trust. It is hoped, by the time we reach adulthood, we will have had the benefit of a mentor in our lives. Mentors in early life appear in many guises: parents, grandparents, teachers, neighbors and heroes and heroines of our youth. They generally have one quality in common: They are able to see that which is unique and special in us. They are the people whose voices echo in the halls of our hearts forever. In *Mentors and Protégés*, Linda Phillips-Jones cites the various types of mentors we may encounter. These include the traditional mentor, generally an older person who helps us develop professionally and achieve career goals.

In *Innovative Teaching Strategies in Nursing*, Barbara Fuszard and Laurie Jowers Taylor describe mentorship as a form of socialization for professional roles, a relationship in which the mentor works closely with the protégé for the purposes of teaching. Mentor behaviors are varied and include teaching new skills and promoting intellectual development, "serving as a guide to enculturate the novice in the values, customs and resources of the profession, serving as a role model, giving advice and counsel during stressful times, assisting the novice in realizing professional goals and aspirations, facilitating the person's advancement in the profession."

Dr. Daniel Levinson gives an interesting view of the mentor. "The mentor takes the younger man (or woman) under his (or her) wing, invites him to a new occupational world, shows him around, imparts his wisdom, cares, sponsors, criticizes and bestows his blessing. The teaching and the sponsoring have their values, but the blessing is the crucial element." (*The Counseling Psychologist*, Vol. 6. No. 1, 1976). In *Passages*, Gail Sheehy refers to Levinson's theory that for a man to achieve success, he needs to have a love relationship and career mentors while in his twenties. Sheehy points out that that kind of relationship would also be beneficial to women.

Although some mentor/protégé relationships seem to happen out of the blue, many are actively sought. Some of the benefits of mentoring relationships include advice on career goals, encouragement, improved skills or knowledge, models to follow, opportunities and resources, and increased exposure and visibility. Linda Philips-Jones identifies steps to finding an appropriate mentor:

1. *Identify your needs.* What is it you hope to gain from the mentoring experience? Are you looking primarily for concrete information and skills? Are you looking for support and direction? Are you trying to gain support within the organization? Are you hopeful that you can effect some change in the organization? This process is useful for two reasons. It helps you clarify your own goals and objectives. You can then, in turn, be clear with your perspective mentor as to what your hopes for the relationship are.
2. *Evaluate yourself as a protégé.* What are your strengths and weaknesses? Are you a pro-active learner? Are you receptive to other people's views? Are you willing to put energy into your learning? A mentor may, in fact, only be as good as his or her protégé. A protégé who is enthusiastic, dedicated and an active learner is almost destined to seek out a teacher who will enhance his or her knowledge. There is truth in the Zen saying, "When the student is ready, the teacher will appear." A true mentor/protégé relationship will have a synergistic quality in which the strengths of each are catalysts for producing new strengths in both.
3. *Begin to identify candidates.* If you are looking for someone to assist you in developing your clinical skills, you will probably want to work with someone whom you admire. Most likely, you will try to find someone with whom you believe you will work well on a personal level.
4. *Develop a plan.* What are your expectations of the mentor? How do you envision the relationship? Do you want to meet on a scheduled

basis? Would you like it to be more informal and open-ended, such as permission to call for advice on various issues? Are you trying to attain a professional credential that has definite requirements, eg, meeting with a superior?

5. *Arrange a meeting.* Here you can give the perspective mentor a plan as to what you hope to accomplish with the relationship, ie, your expectations of the mentor. It may well be that the kind of relationship you propose is suitable for the prospective mentor. Or it may require some negotiation or adjustment so you can determine the starting point for an important and productive relationship.

Where to Begin Your Search

For most people, the most logical and convenient place to begin your search is at your own front door — your own organization. As Phillips-Jones notes, there are various types of mentors. Most probably, especially in the early stages of one's career, one looks for either the traditional mentor (the person who acts as teacher) or the supportive boss. If you are looking for someone who can assist you in developing your clinical skills, look for someone who is experienced and has a high level of skill. This may be difficult to assess, but one indicator is how that person is viewed in the agency and enjoys what he or she does. Another important quality is sensing a mutual compatibility. A mentor may be highly skilled, but if you find it difficult to get along, it can tend to make the relationship much less productive and pleasant.

Organizational Supervisors or Mentors

Some organizations recognize the need for continuing professional growth and supervision and assign a person to provide supervision and allocate agency time for this purpose. They will be people you feel you can learn from. Generally, it is positive to have this sort of arrangement because it facilitates many types of professional licensing requirements and relieves the protégé of much of the guesswork and effort involved in finding his or her own mentor. Because the time is given, mentor and protégé don't need to sacrifice personal time.

Sources Outside the Agency for Mentors

The importance of membership in at least one professional organization cannot be stressed enough. Simply having access to a professional journal can help you see the direction in which the profession is moving and keep you current in the field. Many people believe that involvement in a professional organization is an integral part of moving forward in your profession. For many in home health care, the professional organization offers an invaluable opportunity to network and find a mentor. Increasingly, as agencies employ people on a per-case basis, professional organizations become even more important in preventing professional isolation and providing mentors to newcomers entering the field. At the end of this book, there is a list of professional organizations that can be contacted for additional information.

QUALITIES THAT CAN SCARE OFF PROSPECTIVE MENTORS

Prospective protégés who seem needy may "scare off" potential mentors. Although many talented individuals may welcome the opportunity to be a mentor to someone, typically people do not want to provide psychological counseling. The goal of mentoring is to encourage professional growth, and although mentors may be supportive of protégés during personal crises, the focus of the work is professional. Also, protégés who require a large investment of time may be unrealistic and overwhelming for the mentor.

Possible Detrimental Aspects of Mentoring

Although there are a variety of benefits to be gained from having a mentor, there are also less than positive aspects. The protégé may find that philosophically, he or she is worlds apart from the mentor. The protégé may find that while he is looking for an open, sharing relationship, the mentor may be given more to a dictatorial stance of "I'll talk; you listen." In a relationship that is no longer satisfying, it is best to move on as diplomatically as possible.

A Network of Mentoring Relationships

Typically, when we think of mentors, we tend to think of one person who is pivotal in one's career. Perhaps to look at the mentor/protégé relationship solely in this one-to-one context is to place unnecessary limitations on it. Kathy Kram, who has done a number of studies on the mentor/protégé relationships, suggests it is most beneficial to network to enjoy a number of mentoring relationships. By forming networks of mentoring relationships, protégés can access a variety of skills and various types of mentors. With a network of mentors, it is feasible to have a traditional mentor in one's own agency who helps the protégé hone clinical skills; friends and family who provide emotional support and stability; and people in the higher echelons of the agency or profession who help make important career decisions and help one meet others who can facilitate their professional goals.

In Miscall Zey's *Mentor Programs: Providing the Right Moves*, the seven steps required for developing a mentoring program include deciding who should participate in the program, matching mentor and protégé, determining length and timing of the program, mode and frequency of interaction, and the responsibilities of both mentor and protégé. Mentoring acknowledges the continuously evolving skill of the professional, rather than seeing education and development as terminal.

Mentoring is also healthy and may be a source of a "helper's high" that is as irresistible as the Sirens' call. Whether prompted by daily routine or an altruism like that of Mother Teresa, most caregivers need to participate in or influence the well-being of others. In health care, it is important to remember that caregivers win many of their successes in inches rather than in decisive victories. Working with patients with AIDS, children with cancer, or individuals with chronic obstructive pulmonary disease (COPD), there are days during which we seem to take one step forward and four steps back. The days that could be described, as Ishmael said in *Moby Dick*, as "a damp, drizzly November in my soul," come with the territory.

Slaying the Dragon

Understanding stress and how much one can tolerate without risking one's well-being is paramount for caregivers. Check off the items that pertain to you in the lists below. If you check off more than three of the physical and behavioral signs, your body may be signaling excessive stress. More than three or four emotional signs of stress may indicate high risk as well.

Physical Signs of Stress

1. Frequent heartburn
2. Lack of appetite
3. Excess weight for your age and height
4. High blood pressure
5. Shortness of breath
6. Missed periods or premenstrual tension
7. Dry mouth and throat
8. Heart palpitations or pounding
9. Excessive perspiration

10. Frequent urination
11. Muscle spasms
12. Frequent headaches
13. Alteration of sleep patterns
14. Excessive nervous energy that hinders relaxation
15. Fainting or nausea
16. Feeling of constant fatigue
17. Chronic constipation or diarrhea
18. Feeling of unexplained fullness
19. Inability to cry or sudden crying
20. Sexual dysfunction
21. Susceptibility to colds
22. Rashes
23. Restlessness

Behavioral Signs of Stress

1. Increased smoking or drinking
2. Eating compulsively when a problem arises
3. Clumsiness or being accident-prone
4. Teeth-grinding, foot-tapping, finger-drumming, etc.
5. Trembling or shaking
6. Uncontrolled nervous laughter
7. Difficulty speaking
8. Feeling the need to take medication every day
9. Temper flare-ups
10. Nightmares
11. Mood swings
12. Distrust of people
13. Nagging
14. Negative self-talk
15. Forgetfulness
16. Looking for "magic bullet" or "magic" event as rescue
17. Loss of direction
18. Sense of martyrdom

Emotional Signs of Stress

1. Inability to laugh
2. Financial worries
3. Feeling distressed all the time
4. Boredom resulting in listlessness

5. Exaggerated fears, such as fear of death, disease, heights, storms, confining spaces, etc.
6. Feelings of rejection from family or friends resulting in tendency to withdraw
7. Dread of weekends
8. Pervasive anger toward significant others and co-workers
9. Sense of despair or hopelessness
10. Decreased concentration
11. Feeling alone with your problems and reluctant to discuss them with anyone
12. Resisting help, a vacation or relaxation

Strategies for Preventing and Alleviating Stress

Once you have identified the external-situational and internal-attitudinal stressors that pertain to you and your work, you can decide what needs to be accepted as is and what needs to be changed. Accepting your own limitations and vulnerabilities helps guard against the tendency to please everyone and do everything. Perfectionism may well be thought of as a disease process of which burnout is born. Therefore, a keener awareness of and sensitivity to your individual symptoms of stress may strengthen your ability to regroup and create a more healthful orientation toward life.

Because stress and burnout are closely aligned with withdrawal from activities once enjoyed and isolation from family and friends, see to it that you have a support system in place for yourself. Camaraderie and an accepting environment ease the feelings of fatigue and lack of control and reinforce constructive criticism and suggestions, a positive outlook, and a sense of personal worth and appreciation. Of course, you must first accept the fact that you need help and that you are not left "shipwrecked on a desert isle" with your problems. Recognize that many people need the emotional assistance of peers, mentors and counselors. In the event of overwhelming stress, depression or other debilitating emotional state, the unique human being that is you is not unique at all — perhaps a saving grace of being human in a society that need not be formidable all the time.

Other strategies geared to self-care and burnout prevention include giving yourself credit for what you do, balancing your working life with your personal life, building in "decompression" time (such as walking and meditation), developing an outside interest or hobby that helps you take time off from stress, and developing better physical and mental relaxation techniques.

One of the most effective "stress-busters" is vigorous exercise. Perhaps a health spa or gym where you can learn to do a work-out routine tailored to your needs is a good idea. Or pursue your interest in a sport that affords you a work-out, such as tennis, racquetball, swimming, hiking, bicycling, etc. Personal trainers are usually available at fitness organizations to help you get started.

As you are now probably saying to yourself, "Sure, I'm a real athlete — my job is so strenuous I have no energy left for anything else," remember that a sense of humor is as important a tool as any you use on the job. The idea is not to become an athlete, but rather to blow off all that steam that accumulates in your system because of the demanding nature of your work. Laugh often at how idiotic life seems at times, and how foolishness seems to prevail. As the old song goes, "Life is just a bowl of cherries; don't take it serious, it's too delirious." Certainly the lyricist did not mean ignore the problems and act irresponsibly in the face of danger, but his words may help stop destructive, negative thoughts and set you back on the path to sanity. They also trigger the idea that to feel less stressed, it may be necessary for you to tolerate others as being just as imperfect as you are — truly a happy concept.

A Caregiver's Bill of Rights

There are several versions of the caregiver's bill of rights. The following is a condensation and adaptation that emphasizes the physical, emotional and spiritual needs of those providing any form of care.

1. I have the right to take care of myself without feeling guilty or selfish, because I know one must maintain him- or herself to care effectively for others.
2. I have the right to assess the amount of care I can reasonably provide in one day (or one shift) and to be forgiven the less important tasks that must be eliminated or put off to the next day.
3. I have the right to ask for help from individuals and other resources when I realize that my own efforts are not enough or need bolstering.
4. I have the right to relax and enjoy my life as I see fit when I am not giving care to an ill person.
5. I have the right to my own feelings and emotions, and I am allowed to express myself appropriately.
6. I have the right to refuse to be manipulated by anyone, including my patient.
7. I have the right to be proud of myself for having the strength and courage to offer and give quality care to others.
8. I have the right to receive a salary or other compensation for my work.

9. I have the right to expect the same consideration and acceptance for myself as I give to others for whom I provide care.
10. I have the right to become allied with caregiver and other support groups in which I can find personal solace and learn more about caregiving and self-care.

Summary

- Become attuned to to your own internal signals of stress, such as fatigue, restlessness, depression, short-temperedness. Have a repertoire of measures you can employ for dealing with these symptoms.

- If many of us need to be more assertive, an equal number need to be more supportive. Compliment the positive in other team members.

- The support you give to others multiplies.

- Join professional groups and associations.

- Treat yourself and your colleagues with the same care and consideration with which you treat your clients.

- Relaxation, fun and sharing are as necessary as oxygen.

- Novices are the children of our professional life. We have an obligation to encourage, nurture and give them the benefit of our expertise and experience. Be patient with them. None of us were born healthcare givers, but reached our goal through the efforts of many teachers.

- Our colleagues are our professional family. We owe them support and honesty.

- We are all students, teachers and therapists to each other.

Chapter 8

"It's a Beautiful Day in the Neighborhood": Networking and Resources

"It's a beautiful day in the neighborhood...a neighborly day in the beauty, would you be mine? Could you be mine?"
Fred Rogers, from the theme song of "Mr. Rogers' Neighborhood"

...Do what is impossible, Lord, when (the Senators) have reached the limit of the possible. Help them find consensus when it looks like there is none. Show them that You are not only a God far off and unreal, but a God who is near, available, and relevant to practical affairs....
Dr. Richard C. Halverson, Chaplain, United States Senate, November 4, 1985

'Tis not enough to help the feeble up, But to support him after.
William Shakespeare, *Timon of Athens*

A student nurse on psychiatric clinical rotation walked into the small conference room. She followed two psychiatrists, three nurses, a social worker, a nurse's aide, two attendants, the ward secretary and a dietitian. The group began to discuss various patients in their charge—how they were doing, any new developments, insights or problems, what they said, what they ate. Listening carefully to all the "testimony," the student found the group's interaction fascinating. Then one of the nurses, who knew to which patients the student nurse had been assigned, asked her what she had observed during her brief tenure with some of the patients. Everyone turned to her and gave her full attention. Not expecting to participate but simply to observe, she added her "testimony" with delight and gratitude. How terrific it was to be only a student, yet be given the floor as a bona fide member of the health care team.

There is a kind of power, she thought even after she became a
registered psychiatric nurse, generated by professionals who consider
and care about what their colleagues think. Caregivers who make
themselves available to other caregivers establish a support system and
networking potential, two factors necessary for personal growth in one's
chosen field.

In addition to staff meetings, charting and other interstaff communications related to the home care of a patient, there are local, state,
national and international organizations that offer information, support
and advice. Professional and nonprofessional caregivers may find the
following list helpful.

The Community at Large

- **Medicare:** 70 percent of patients treated by home health agencies
  are older than 65. Medicare, the national health care program for the
  elderly, may be the primary insurance for these patients. Age is the
  criterion of eligibility. Typically, Medicare pays 80 percent of what
  are considered reasonable costs.
- **Medicaid:** a national, means-tested health care program to help poor
  people pay for doctors and hospital costs. There are differences in
  what charges Medicaid and Medicare will reimburse. Typically, both
  programs reimburse for home health services. Call the programs' 800
  numbers for booklets detailing services and costs.
- **Private insurance companies:** free agents whose coverage may or
  may not include home health services. Insurance needs to be checked
  by calling the company directly. Many of elderly people carry
  supplemental policies in addition to Medicare. It is rare for these
  policies to pay for home health services beyond what Medicare will
  cover.
- **The United Way:** a national organization whose mission is to
  organize local funding efforts. Many United Way chapters publish
  what is known as the "Red Book," a comprehensive list of local
  social organizations and their functions. The list is tremendously
  helpful to health care workers in locating services for their patients.
- **American Cancer Society** (ACS): a national organization with
  many local chapters. ACS, an important resource for cancer patients
  and their families, provides general information on education,
  support groups, community resources, equipment, etc. Varying
  stipends may be available for uncovered cancer-related expenses.
- **Office on Aging:** local offices that help with information on what
  services are available for seniors.

Local Organizations

- **County Board of Social Services:** local administrators of a variety of federal means-tested programs, such as AFDC (Aid to Families with Dependent Children), Medicaid, and special Medicaid programs.
- **Local senior centers:** community-operated centers that offer social activities, dances, educational lectures, workshops and health screenings, lunch programs, and information on other services for the elderly. A center may also have volunteers who assist seniors with medical bill payment. Some senior centers have caregiver seminars that educate significant others on the availability of resources.
- **The Salvation Army**: an international religious and charitable group, organized along military lines, founded in 1878 by William Booth. The Salvation Army is actively involved in a variety of social service activities in many American communities. Best known for its soup kitchens and food pantries, the Army also has hospitals, social service organizations and alcohol and drug rehabilitation centers. Members are well-qualified to give information on where to find other community services.
- **Religious organizations:** churches, synagogues, temples and religious communities may offer a variety of programs and services. While many are involved in social service, these services are highly individualized and vary considerably. One church might offer rides to physician's appointments or shopping, whereas another will operate a food pantry. Health care workers need to know members of the organizations. Some organizations are also helpful in locating translators when one encounters a language barrier.
- **Police department:** the law-enforcement team that can provide escort services in dangerous areas, if the home health agency has not hired someone to do this, provide information on types of crimes being committed in certain areas, offer knowledge of state laws, etc. In most communities, police must be notified of hospice cases, and, in some states, view a patient who has died.
- **Protective services:** organizations that insure protection of those who may be at a disadvantage in advocating for themselves— including the elderly, the physically handicapped, or developmentally delayed. Staff will investigate situations that pose a threat to these individuals.
- **Postal workers**: civil servants employed by the United States Postal Service. Because the mail carrier may be the only person who has daily contact with the patient or the patient's residence, he or she

may be a valuable resource as to the well-being of people in the community.

- **Pharmacies and equipment companies**: operations from the "Mom and Pop" corner drug store to the multimillion-dollar businesses that may provide effective products and services. Find the efficient ones in your community. It will save you and your patient time and frustration.
- **Fraternal organizations:** clubs and associations (Elks, Moose, Kiwanis, Rotary, etc.) that undertake some form of community service, such as raising funds for charities, supplying equipment (beds and wheelchairs), and providing eyeglasses to volunteers.
- **First-aid squads:** local volunteers called on to transport people who are suddenly taken ill to the hospital emergency room or other facility for medical care. The first-aid squad may also transport patients to or from the hospital. Team members are usually trained in CPR and other emergency measures.
- **Meals on Wheels:** a meal program funded by state and county grants that has long delivered hot meals to homebound persons who are unable to care for themselves. Manned by volunteers from the community, Meals on Wheels is an invaluable resource for the homebound person. There may be a waiting list and financial eligibility requirements.
- **Maternal Child Health Clinics:** programs run by community agencies such as the Visiting Nurse Association that provide clinical and social services to mothers and children.

State, National and International Resources

Aging Network Services (for geriatric care managers)
4400 East-West Hwy., Suite 907
Bethesda, MD 20814
(301) 657-4329

AIDS Health Project
P.O. Box 0884
San Francisco, CA 94143-0884
(415) 476-6430

Al-Anon Family Group Headquarters (alcoholism)
P.O. Box 862,
Midtown Station
New York, NY 10018
(800) 433-2666

Allergy and Asthma Network
(Mothers of Asthmatics, Inc.)
3554 Chain Bridge Road, Suite 200
Fairfax, VA 22030-2709
(703) 385-4403

Alzheimer's Disease & Related Disorders Association
919 N. Michigan Avenue, Suite 1000
Chicago, IL 60611
(800) 272-3900

American Amputee Foundation
P.O. Box 250218, Hillcrest Station
Little Rock, AR 72225
(501) 666-2523

American Anorexia-Bulimia Association
c/o Regents Hospital
425 East 61st Street, 6th Floor
New York, NY 10021
(212) 891-8686

American Association of Homes and Services for the Aging
901 E Street N.W., Suite 500
Washington, DC 20004
(202) 783-2242

American Association of Kidney Patients
100 South Ashley Drive, Suite 280
Tampa, FL 33602
(800) 749-2257

American Association on Mental Retardation
444 North Capitol Street, N.W., Suite 846
Washington, DC 20001
(202) 387-1968

American Association of Occupational Health Nurses (AAOHN)
3500 Piedmont Road N.E.
Atlanta, GA 30305-1315

American Association for Respiratory Care
11030 Ables Lane
Dallas, TX 75229-4593
(214) 243-2272

American Association of Retired Persons (AARP)
601 E Street N.W.
Washington, DC 20049
(202) 434-2277

American Cancer Society   1599 Clifton Road
777 Third Avenue   Atlanta, GA 30331
New York, NY 10017   (800) ACS-2345
(212) 371-2900

American College of Nurse Midwives (ACNM)
1522 K Street, N.W., Suite 1120
Washington, DC 20005

American Council of the Blind
1155 15th Street N.W., Suite 720
Washington, DC 20005
(800) 424-8666

American Chronic Pain Association
P.O. Box 850
Rocklin, CA 95677
(916) 632-0922

American Deafness and Rehabilitation Association
P.O. Box 251554
Little Rock, AR 72225
(501) 868-8850

American Diabetes Association (ADA)
1660 Duke Street
Alexandria, VA 22314
(800) 323-3472

American Federation of Home Health Agencies
1320 Fenwick Lane, Suite 100
Silver Spring, MD 20910
(301) 588-1454

American Foundation for the Blind
15 West 16th Street
New York, NY 10011
(800) 232-5463

American Foundation for Urologic Disease, Inc.
300 West Pratt Street, Suite 401
Baltimore, MD 21201 - 2463
(410) 727-2908

American Heart Association
7272 Greenville Avenue
Dallas, TX 75231
(214) 373-6300

American Holistic Nurses Association (AHNA)
Box 116
Telluride, CO 81435

American Institute for Cancer Research
1759 R Street N.W.
Washington, DC 20009
(800) 843-8114

American Kidney Fund
6110 Executive Blvd., Suite 1010
Rockville, MD 20852
(800) 638-8299

American Liver Foundation
1425 Pompton Avenue
Cedar Grove, NJ 07009
(201) 256-2550

American Lung Association
1740 Broadway
New York, NY 10019
(212) 315 - 8700

American Lupus Society
3914 Del Amo Blvd., Suite 922
Torrance, CA 90503
(310) 542 - 8891

American Nurses' Association (ANA)
2420 Pershing Road
Kansas City, MO 64108

American Occupational Therapy Association
4720 Montgomery Lane
P.O. Box 31220
Bethesda, MD 20824-1220
(301) 652-2682

American Paralysis Foundation (spinal cord injury)
500 Morris Avenue
Springfield, NJ 07081
(800) 225-0292

American Parkinson Disease Association
60 Bay Street, Suite 401
Staten Island, NY 10301
(800) 223-2732

American Physical Therapy Association
1111 North Fairfax Street
Alexandria, VA 22314
(703) 684-2782

American Psychiatric Association
1400 K Street, N.W.
Washington, DC 20005-2492
(202) 682-6000

American Public Health Association (APHA)
Public Health Nursing Section
1015 15th Street, N.W.
Washington, DC 20005

American Social Health Association (sexually transmitted diseases)
P.O. Box 13827
Research Triangle Park, NC 27709
(919) 361-8400

Amyotrophic Lateral Sclerosis Association ("Lou Gehrig's disease")
21021 Ventura Blvd., Suite 321
Woodland Hills, CA 91364
(800) 782-4747

Andrus Gerontology Center
University of Southern California
University Park, MC 0191
Los Angeles, CA 90089
(213) 740-6060

Aplastic Anemia Foundation of America
P.O. Box 22689
Baltimore, MD 21203
(410) 955-2803

Arthritis Foundation
1314 Spring Street, N.W.
Atlanta, GA 30309
(800) 283-7800

Association of Pediatric Oncology Nurses (APON)
5000 Birch, P.O. Box 2690 - 175
Newport Beach, CA 92660

Association for Practitioners in Infection Control (APIC)
505 E. Hawley
Mundelein, IL 60060

Association of Rehabilitation Nurses (ARN)
2506 Gross Point Road
Evanston, IL 60201

AT&T Accessible Communications Product Center 5
Woodhollow Road, Room 1119
Parsippany, NJ 07054
(800) 233 - 1222
(800) 233 - 3232 (TDD)

Cancer Care
1180 Avenue of the Americas
New York, NY 10036
(212) 221 - 3300

Cancer Information Service
Building 31, Room 10A-07
9000 Rockville Pike
Bethesda, MD 20892
(301) 496 - 8664

Canine Companions for Independence
P.O. Box 446
Santa Rosa, CA 95402-0446
(707) 528-0830

Caretenders Health Corp. (products and services for seniors)
9200 Shelbyville Road, Suite 810
Louisville, KY 40222
(800) 845-6987

Center for Disease Control and Prevention (CDC)
1600 Clifton Road, N.E.
Atlanta, GA 30333
(404) 639-3311

Center for Disease Control and Prevention National AIDS
Clearinghouse
P.O. Box 6003
Rockville, MD 20849-6003
(800) 458-5231

Center for Family Support (mentally disabled)
386 Park Avenue South, Suite 1201
New York, NY 10016
(212) 889-5464

Chemotherapy Foundation
183 Madison Avenue, Room 403
New York, NY 10016
(212) 213-9292

Children of Aging Parents
609 Woodbourne, Suite 302-A
Levittown, PA 19057
215) 345-5104

Children's Blood Foundation (CBF)
333 East 38th Street, Suite 830
New York, NY 10016
(212) 297-4336

Choice in Dying
200 Varick Street, Suite 1001
New York, NY 10014-4810
(800) 989-9455

Council on Family Health
225 Park Avenue South, Suite 1700
New York, NY 10003 (212) 598-3617

Crohn's Disease and Colitis Foundation of America, Inc.
386 Park Avenue South
New York, NY 10016
(212) 685-3440

Cystic Fibrosis Foundation
6931 Arlington Road
Bethesda, MD 20814
(800) FIGHT CF or (301) 951-4422

Deafness Research Foundation
9 East 38th Street
New York, NY 10016
(800) 535-3323

Digestive Disease National Coalition
711 Second Street, N.E., Suite 200
Washington, DC 20002
(202) 544-7497

Epilepsy Foundation of America
4351 Garden City Drive
Landover, MD 20785
(800) 332-1000

Family Service America
11700 West Lake Park Drive
Milwaukee, WI 53224
(414) 359-1040

Family Medical Pharmacy
839 South Harbor Boulevard
Anaheim, CA 92085
(714) 722-4840

Foundation for Hospice & Home Care
519 C Street N.E.
Washington, DC 20002
(202) 547-6586

Health Education Resource Organization (HERO)
101 West Reed Street, Suite
825 Baltimore, MD 21201
(410) 685-1180

Hearlog Aid Helpline
20361 Middlebelt Road
Livonia, MI 48152
(800) 521-5247

Hearing Helpline Better Hearing Institute
P.O. Box 1840
Washington, DC 20013
(800) 327-9355

Chapter 8

Help for Incontinent People
P.O. Box 544
Union, SC 29379
(803) 579-7900

High Blood Pressure Information Center
National Institutes of Health
4733 Bethesda Avenue
Bethesda, MD 20814
(301) 952-3260

Health Insurance Association of America
1025 Connecticut Avenue N.W.
Washington, DC 20036
(800) 277-4486

Home Care Council of New Jersey
201 Bloomfield Avenue, Suite 3
Verona, NJ 07044
(201) 857-3333

Huntington's Disease Society of America
140 West 22nd Street, 6th Floor
New York, NY 10011-2420
(800) 345-4372

International Association for the Study of Pain
909 NE 43rd Street, Suite 306
Seattle, WA 98105-6020
(206) 547-6409

International Association of Laryngectomees
1599 Clifton Road, N.E.
Atlanta, GA 30029-4251
(404) 329-7651

Juvenile Diabetes Foundation International
432 Park Avenue South
New York, NY 10016-8013
(800) 533-2873

Kelly Assisted Living
P.O. Box 331180
Detroit, MI 48232
(800) 541-9818

Leukemia Society of America
600 Third Avenue, 4th Floor
New York, NY 10016
(212) 573-8484

Look Good, Feel Better (LGFB)
(Cosmetic, Toiletry, and Fragrance Association Foundation)
1101 17th Street, N.W., Suite 300
Washington, DC 20036
(202) 331-1770

Lupus Foundation
Four Research Place, Suite 180
Rockville, MD 20850-3226
(301) 670-9292

Maddak, Inc. (products and aids for daily living)
6 Industrial Road
Pequannock, NJ 07470
(800) 443-4926

Make-A-Wish Foundation of America
100 West Claringdon Avenue, Suite 2200
Phoenix, AZ 85013
(602) 279-9474

Make Today Count
101 1/2 South Union Street
Alexandria, VA 22314-3323
(703) 548-9674

March of Dimes Defects Foundation
1275 Mamaroneck Avenue
White Plains, NY 10605
(914) 428-7100

Maxi Aids
(visually, hearing and physically impaired)
P.O. Box 3209
Farmingdale, NY 11735
(800) 522-6294
(714) 846-4799 in New York

Medic Alert Foundation International
P.O. Box 1009
Turlock, CA 95381-1009
(209) 668-3333

Medicare address according to zip code
(800) 638-6833

M&M Health Care Apparel Co.
1541 60th Street
Brooklyn, NY 11219
(800) 221-8929

Muscular Dystrophy Association
330 East Sunrise Drive
Tucson, AZ 85718
(602) 529-2000

Myasthenia Gravis Foundation
222 S. Riverside Plaza, Suite
1540 Chicago, IL 60606
(800) 541-5454

National Association for Practical Nurse Education and Service
(NAPNES)
10801 Pear Tree Lane, Suite 151
St. Louis, MO 63074

National Association on Drug Abuse Problems
355 Lexington Avenue, 2nd Floor
New York, NY 10017-6683
(212) 986-1170

National Association for Home Care
519 C Street, N.E.
Washington, DC 20002-5809
(202) 547-7424

National Association of People with AIDS (NAPWA)
1413 K Street, N.W.
Washington, DC 20005
(202) 898-0414

National Association for Sickle Cell Disease
3345 Wilshire Boulevard, Suite 1106
Los Angeles, CA 90010-1880
(213) 736-5455

National Chronic Pain Outreach Association (NCPOA)
7979 Old Georgetown Road, Suite 100
Bethesda, MD 20814-2429
(301) 652-4948

National Coalition of Hispanic Health & Human Services
1502 16th Street, N.W.
Washington, DC 20036
(202) 387-5000

National Committee on the Treatment of Intractable Pain
c/o Wayne Coy, Jr.
Cohn and Marks
1333 New Hampshire Avenue, N.W
Washington, DC 20036
(202) 452-4836

National Council on Aging
409 3rd Street SW., Suite 200
Washington, DC 20024
(800) 424-9046

National Council on Alcoholism
1511 K Street, N.W.
Washington, DC
(800) 622-2255

National Digestive Diseases Information Clearinghouse
P.O. Box NDDIC
9000 Rockville Pike
Bethesda, MD 20892
(301) 468-6344

National Down's Syndrome Congress
1605 Chantilly Drive, Suite 250
Atlanta, GA 30324
(404) 633-1555

National Easter Seal Society
230 West Monroe Street, Suite 1800
Chicago, IL 60606
(312) 726-6200

National Federation of Interfaith Volunteer Caregivers, Inc.
368 Broadway, Suite 105
Kingston, NY 12401
(914) 331-1198

National Foundation for Ileitis & Colitis, Inc.
444 Park Avenue South, 11th Floor
New York, NY 10018
(800) 343-3637

Chapter 8

National Head Injury Foundation
1776 Massachusetts Avenue, N.W., Suite 100
Washington, DC 20036
(202) 296-6443

National Health Information Center
U.S. Department of Health & Human Services
P.O. Box 1133
Washington, DC 20013
(800) 336-4797

National Heart, Lung, and Blood Institute (NHLBI) Information
Center
P.O. Box 30105
Bethesda, MD 20824-0105
(301) 251-1222

National Hemophilia Foundation (NHF)
110 Green Street, Suite 303
New York, NY 10012
(212) 219-8180

National Hospice Organization
1901 North Moore Street, Suite 901
Arlington, VA 22209
(800) 658-8898

National Hypertension Association, Inc.
324 East 30th Street
New York, NY 10016
(212) 889-3557

National Institute of Neurological Disorders and Stroke
9000 Rockville Pike
Building 31, Room 8A-06
Bethesda, MD 20892
(301) 496-5751

National Jewish Center for Immunology and Respiratory Medicine
1400 Jackson Street
Denver, CO 80206
(303) 388-4461

National Kidney Foundation
30 East 33rd Street, Suite 1100
New York, NY 10016
(212) 889-2210

National Leukemia Association
585 Stewart Avenue, Suite 536
Garden City, NY 11530
(516) 222-1944

National Lymphedema Network (NLN)
2211 Post Street, Suite 404
San Francisco, CA 94115
(800) 541-3259

National Marrow Donor Program
3433 Broadway, N.E., Suite 400
Minneapolis, MN 55413
(612) 627-5800

National Mental Health Association
1021 Prince Street
Alexandria, VA 22314-2971
(703) 684-7722

National Multiple Sclerosis Society
733 3rd Avenue, 6th Floor
New York, NY 10017
(800) 344-4867 or (800) 532-7667

National Organization for Rare Disorders
P.O. Box 8923
New Fairfield, CT 06812
(800) 999-6673

National Osteoporosis Foundation
1150 17th Street, N.W., Suite 500
Washington, DC 20036
(202) 223-2226

National Parkinson Foundation
1502 N.W. 9th Avenue
Miami, FL 33136
(800) 327-4545

National Rehabilitation Information Center
8455 Colesville Road, Suite 935
Silver Spring, MD 20910
(800) 346-2742

National Stroke Association
8480 East Orchard Road, Suite 1000
Englewood, CO 80111-5015
(303) 762-9922

Nutrition Education Association
P.O. Box 20301
3647 Glan Haven
Houston, TX 77225
(713) 665-2946

Occupational Safety and Health Administration (OSHA)
U.S. Department of Labor
200 Constitution Avenue, N.W.
Washington, DC 20210
(202) 219-8148

Pediatric AIDs Foundation
1311 Colorado Avenue
Santa Monica, CA 90404
(310) 395-9051

Phoenix Society for Burn Survivors (PSBS)
11 Rust Hill Road
Levittown, PA 19056
(215) 946-BURN

Self-Help Clearinghouse
St. Claire's Riverside Medical Center
Pocono Road
Denville, NJ 07834
(201) 625-7101

Simon Foundation for Continence
P.O. Box 835
Wilmette, IL 60091
(708) 864 - 3913

Skin Cancer Foundation
245 Fifth Avenue, Suite 2402
New York, NY 10016
(212) 725 - 5176

Social Security (Address according to zip code)
(800) 772 - 1213

Thyroid Foundation of America
Ruth Sleeper Hall, Room 350 40
Parkman Street
Boston, MA 02114-1202
(617) 726-8500

United Cerebral Palsy Association
1522 K Street, N.W., Suite 1112
Washington, DC 20005
(202) 842 - 1266

United Ostomy Association
35 Executive Park, Suite 120
Irvine, CA 92714
(714) 660-8624

United Scleroderma Foundation
P.O. Box 399
Watsonville, CA 95077
(800) 722-4673

Visiting Nurse Association of America
3801 East Florida Avenue, Suite 900
Denver, CO 80210
800) 426-2547

Summary

The Community at Large:

- Medicare: 70 percent of patients treated by home health agencies are older than 65. Medicare, the national health care program for the elderly, may be the primary insurance for these patients. Age is the criterion of eligibility. Typically, Medicare pays 80 percent of what are considered reasonable costs.

- Medicaid: a national, means-tested health care program to help poor people pay for doctors and hospital costs.

- There are differences in what charges Medicaid and Medicare will reimburse. Typically, both programs reimburse for home health services. Call the programs' 800 numbers for booklets detailing services and costs.

- Private insurance companies: free agents whose coverage may or may not include home health services. Insurance needs to be checked by calling the company directly. Many elderly people carry supplemental policies in addition to Medicare. It is rare for these policies to pay for home health services beyond what Medicare will cover.

- The United Way: a national organization whose mission is to organize local funding efforts. Many United Way chapters publish what is known as the "Red Book," a comprehensive list of local social organizations and their functions. The list is tremendously helpful to health care workers in locating services for their patients.

- American Cancer Society: a national organization with many local chapters. ACS, an important resource for cancer patients and their families, provides general information on education, support groups, community resources, equipment, etc. Varying stipends may be available for uncovered cancer-related expenses.

- Office on Aging: local offices that help with information on what services are available for seniors.

Local Organizations:
- County Board of Social Services: local administrators of a variety of federal means-tested programs, such as AFDC (Aid to Families with Dependent Children), Medicaid and special Medicaid programs.

- Local senior centers: community operated centers that offer social activities, dances, educational lectures, workshops and health screenings, trips, lunch programs, and information on other services for the elderly. A center may also have volunteers who assist seniors with medical bill payment. Some senior centers have caregiver seminars that educate significant others on the availability of resources.

- The Salvation Army: an international religious and charitable group organized along military lines, founded in 1878 by William Booth. The Salvation Army is actively involved in a variety of social service activities in many American communities. Best known for its soup kitchens and food pantries, the Army also has hospitals, social service organizations, and drug and alcohol rehab centers. Members are well qualified to give information on where to locate other community services.

- Religious organizations: churches, synagogues, temples and religious communities may offer a variety of programs and services. While many are involved in social service, these services are highly individualized and vary considerably. One church might offer rides to physician appointments or shopping, whereas another will operate a food pantry. Health care workers need to know members of the organizations. Some organizations are helpful in locating translators when one encounters a language barrier.

- Police department: the law enforcement team in each community that can provide escort services in dangerous areas, if the agency has not hired someone to do this, provide information on types of crimes being committed in certain areas, offer knowledge of state laws, etc. In most communities, police must be notified of hospice cases, and in some states, must view a patient who has died.

- Protective services: organizations that insure protection of those who may be at a disadvantage in advocating for themselves---including the elderly, the physically handicapped, or developmentally disabled. Staff will investigate situations that pose a threat to these individuals.

- Postal workers: civil servants employed by the United States Postal Service. Because the mail carrier may be the only person who has daily contact with the patient or a patient's residence, he or she may be a valuable resource as to the well-being of people in the community.

- Pharmacies and equipment companies: operations from the "Mom and Pop" corner drug store to multimillion dollar businesses that may provide effective services or products. Find the efficient ones in your community. It will save you and your patient time and frustration.

- Fraternal organizations: clubs and associations that undertake some form of community service, such as raising funds for charities, supplying equipment (beds, wheelchairs), and providing eyeglasses to volunteers.

- First-aid squads: local volunteers who are on call to transport people who have suddenly taken ill to the hospital emergency room or other facility for medical care. The first-aid squad may also transport patients to or from the hospital. Team members are usually trained in CPR and other emergency measures.

- Meals on Wheels: a meal program funded by state and county grants that has long delivered hot meals to homebound persons who are unable to care for themselves. Manned by volunteers from the community, Meals on Wheels is an invaluable resource for the homebound person. There may be a waiting list and financial eligibility requirements.

- Maternal Child Health Clinics: programs run by community agencies such as Visiting Nurse Associations that provide clinical and social services to mothers and children.

"Safe Home": Safety and Liability Issues

Better safe (or sure) than sorry.
(19th-century proverb)

A man surprised is half beaten.
(French proverb)

Ignorance of the law excuses no man.
John Selden, 17th-century
English jurist

Martha Ballard, a midwife/healer between 1785 and 1812, assisted at 816 births in the Hallowell, Maine, area. She kept a diary of her work, an important legacy bearing a message for anyone who approaches another person's home with the intention of providing care.

> *"[April 24] A* sever Storm of rain. I was Calld at 1 hour pm from Mrs Husseys by Ebenzer Hewin. Crosst the river in their Boat. A great sea A going. We got safe over then sett out for Mr Hewins. I Crost a stream, on the way on fleeting Loggs & got safe over. Wonder full is the Goodness of providence. I then proceeded on my journey. Went beyond Mr Hainses & a Larg tree blew up by the roots before me which Caused my hors to spring back & my life was spared. Great & marvillous are thy sparing mercies O God. I was assisted over the fallen tree by Mr Hains. Went on. Soon Came to a stream. The Bridg was gone. Mr Hewin took the rains waded thro & led the horse. Assisted by the same allmighty power I got safe thro & arivd unhurt. Mrs Hewins safe delivd at 10 h Evn of a Daughter."
> ---from *A Midwife's Tale* by Laurel Thatcher Ulrich

Every health-caregiver owes it to him- or herself to be as safe as possible and to understand how laws of the county, state and federal government, policies of the health care agency or facility, and tenets of one's specific occupation affect daily work with patients. At times, home health caregivers may feel they, like Martha Ballard, must battle the elements and cope with hardships. Luckily, however, our age of information, technology and convenience affords us some "marvillous sparing mercies" Ballard never dreamed of. We've come a long way from packing ourselves onto a horse to get to a patient's home. Our storms and raging rivers instead seem to manifest in the form of powerful diseases and human limits.

But health care has been and continues to be studied, so the human limits have become fewer. Undoubtedly, scientists and sages proclaim, the best cure for any ill-being is prevention. Prevention rises to the most exalted position in issues of personal and legal safety, from avoiding infection and contamination to preventing a fire in a patient's home, from taking action that is known to be acceptable according to the law to carrying adequate malpractice insurance.

According to William Foege, MD, of The Carter Center in Atlanta, Ga., infectious diseases and violence are two factors that continue to pose public health concern. In an article in the 1995 annual *Contempo* issue of the *Journal of the American Medical Association* (JAMA), Foege writes: "Infectious disease control was once synonymous with public health. The decreasing role it played as chronic diseases, environmental, and occupational health problems were expanding is being reversed." He continues by warning that knowledge of a disease doesn't necessarily guarantee eradication. He cites AIDS as an example, saying that we know how to prevent AIDS transmission, but the ineffectual use of that knowledge will result in transmission.

Foege also cites violence as an evolving theme in the public health arena. Only a decade ago, violence was frequently dismissed as a public health problem. Addressing changes in the field, Foege says a broader, more accurate definition of violence is coming into use, going beyond the obvious physical trauma to include mental violence, fear, and psychological trauma. He writes that low- and high-technology approaches are being suggested to make handguns as childproof as aspirin bottles, to personalize handguns so they can be shot only by the owners, and to hold responsible both the trigger "pullers" and the trigger "makers."

Furthermore, Foege declares that the practice of public health is changing beyond any predictions and that there have been significant strides in public attitudes and policies. However, he writes: "The antigovernment mood, more obvious in the past year, leads to fears of a reduction in government support for public health."

When the Patient is Suicidal

It is incredibly tragic when we read of someone who has died as a result of abuse, self-neglect or suicide. We ask ourselves why wasn't someone there and couldn't they have done something to prevent this. In the case of the home-care patient, we will be the ones who will be there, and it will be up to us to do something.

There are a variety of factors that may place a home-care patient at high risk for suicide, a form of violence turned against oneself. They include the trauma of the illness itself, multiple or concurrent losses in the patient's own life, or possibly adverse reactions to medications. *When a person makes a statement that he or she will commit suicide, it must always be taken seriously.* Certainly, statements of this type must be reported to a supervisor. A variety of elements need to be explored, usually by a social worker or psychiatric nurse:

- the rationality of the patient
- disturbances in thought processes
- the person's history of depression or psychiatric illness
- other suicide attempts
- a precipitating event
- a patient's expressed plan to commit suicide
- lack of persons supportive of the patient
- a patient's isolation
- medication difficulties

The team member will need to be assured that the person will not act on his or her ideation of suicide.

Perhaps the best advice for caregivers who work in the clients' homes is to familiarize yourself with every possible means of protection from medical and non-medical difficulties that may arise.

Medical Protection

1. Never—ever—become lackadaisical about preventive measures because you think the patient looks "like such a nice person" or you think you couldn't possibly "catch" anything because you're tough or of resilient stock.
2. Use gloves whenever you are performing a task that may possibly involve direct skin contact with a patient's bodily fluids or secretions.

3. Teach your patient to cover his mouth with tissue or a paper towel when he coughs or sneezes and to discard the tissue directly into a container with a lid.
4. Understand how a particular disease may be transmitted to others and avoid coming into contact with any means of transmission.
5. Be careful about hugging a patient. It may be instinctive for you, but even a fleeting moment of close contact with a patient with an infectious illness could be a disaster.
6. If you are in a seriously fatigued, weakened or stressed state, call in sick or take extra measures to protect yourself from infection. Use all preventive measures available, such as wearing a surgical mask, gloves and gown. Signs of "coming down with something" or feeling extremely stressed may increase your susceptibility to disease.
7. Seek immunizations, such as the Hepatitis B vaccine, through your agency, facility, clinic or physician.
8. Participate in health screenings, such as those for hypertension and tuberculosis.
9. Encourage good ventilation in the patient's home, if possible.
10. Encourage moderate temperature as well. An environment that is too warm may help incubate germs, and one that is too cold may cause stress and discomfort.
11. Do not eat food handed to you by your patient. Do not eat off a patient's tray or dish. Do not drink from any cup or glass your patient uses.
12. Wash your hands, wrists and forearms often and thoroughly with plenty of soap and hot water. If you cannot wash in a patient's residence, carry moist towelettes and alcohol wipes. Everyone, no matter what her job title, should make handwashing a priority at least before and after contact with a patient.
13. Your uniform or the clothing you wear when on duty with your patients should be laundered daily.
14. Do not sit on a patient's bed.
15. Employ good body mechanics when moving or lifting a patient.
16. Make sure the patient's kitchen, bathroom, commode and other personal facilities are kept scrupulously clean.
17. Learn the proper way to dispose of medical or contaminated waste.
18. Keep your hands away from your mouth, nose and eyes while in a client's home. Before you use the toilet, wash your hands. Germs may enter the body through the genital area. And wash your hands after using the toilet.
19. If the patient's home is infested with insects or rodents, ask for an exterminator. Bugs may carry "bugs."

20. Disinfect the patient's telephone receiver—earpiece and mouthpiece —with alcohol wipes or similar product. Using a telephone an infected patient held to his ear and mouth may be risky.
21. Eat well, sleep well, exercise, think positively and meditate. The better you take care of yourself, the more effective your immune system will be.
22. Wash and/or disinfect all devices and equipment your patient touched during your session. You don't want germs to spread to you or other clients.
23. Touching a client is often considered therapeutic and caring, but be mindful of the gestures. Avoid kissing your patients and their significant others. A pat on the arm may be preferable to a handshake.
24. Avoid touching wound dressings, etc., unless part of your job requires that you do and you proceed safely. A physical therapist, occupational therapist, homemaker, chaplain or other caregiver *not* required to perform medical or nursing care should not touch skin that has a rash, for example.
25. If a patient has pets, be relatively certain they are not a source of transmission or contamination. Beware of even the friendliest little dog who sits all day with a patient and licks his face and hands.

Non-medical Protection

Many years ago, before there were standard mechanisms in place for protective services and home-care policies to prevent mishaps and disasters for caregivers, a registered nurse who mostly did private duty recounts a story involving two different types of safety issues.

"I took care of a wealthy woman in a rich neighborhood in Newark, NJ. Her daughter went out shopping each day and always left the doors open. I was asked to leave the door open for the daughter when she returned home. However, since I had read about a robbery in that same neighborhood, I was frightened to leave the door unlocked. So I locked the door after the daughter had left and then had to continuously watch to see when she drove her car up to the house. Then I quickly unlocked the door before she got to it. It was quite nerve-racking.

With this same patient, I had to get into the stall shower to assist her while I gave her a shower. She was unable to stand very long and needed to be held for support. I didn't stay on this case too long."

A far grimmer story, of visiting nurse Marcia Granucci, 45, appeared on page one of the Asbury Park Press on November 18, 1995. Employed by a VNA, Ms. Granucci went on a Thursday afternoon to visit her patients, an 85-year-old man and his 89-year-old wife in West Long Branch, NJ.

According to the newspaper report, Ms. Granucci walked in as the couple's 54-year-old son shot his parents to death. He then shot her and himself. The three dead bodies were discovered just after noon on Friday; the gunman died from his wounds on Sunday. Ms. Granucci left behind her husband, two teenaged children, friends, relatives and traumatized home health professionals. The feature story that focused on the nurse included the following statement:

> "Nursing officials interviewed yesterday acknowledged that danger is part of the job. Granucci knew that, too, as do thousands of nurses who every day knock on the doors of strangers' houses not knowing who is on the other side.... Nurses and others who care for the sick have to make those choices, especially as the country moves more toward home health care...."

Today, health caregivers must establish a plan of care that is beneficial to the patient as well as reasonable for the caregiver. A social worker tells of one of her clients, a woman with muscular dystrophy who lived alone in a senior housing building. Although only in her late 50s, the woman had physically deteriorated to the point that she could not press a button or lift the phone. She was extremely vulnerable, nearly helpless except for her sharp mind, and she insisted on remaining in her apartment.

Her several caregivers included her boyfriend and her sister, who erratically came and went, a nurse and assistive personnel. The woman often accused the caregivers of stealing her valuables; she became increasingly difficult and manipulative. When she demanded that the nurse hold the key to her apartment so she could let herself in each day, the nurse said she preferred that someone meet her at the woman's apartment to let her in. The home-health agency policy opposed a caregiver's possessing a key to anyone's home.

However, the woman's boyfriend and sister pressed the nurse to keep the key. This inappropriate responsibility caused her a good deal of trepidation, and she suggested to her agency supervisor that perhaps in this case her services should not be provided. The supervisor insisted, according to the agency's mission, that care be provided regardless of adversarial conditions. But at least the nurse acquired the support of her agency and protective services, who were notified that care was being provided under duress. A caregiver of any discipline should:

a.   immediately notify the appropriate persons of the problem or a potential problem and discuss the possible solutions, and
b.   promptly document the notification and discussions.

Keep Fear from Defeating Your Health Care

Other non-medical protection involves preventing hazards and knowing in advance what to do in case of an emergency. The major hazards include fire, loss of electricity or water supply, telephone malfunction, dangerous conditions caused by weather, car breakdown, property negligence such as broken stairs, windows, doors, appliances, etc., and rodent and insect infestation. The following suggestions may help the caregiver avoid difficulties or deal with them successfully.

1.   Cooking, smoking, poor wiring and electrical devices, fireplace usage and flammable substances cause most house fires. Check a client's smoking habits and create safer circumstances—ashtrays, supervision of client and others when using matches and lighters, etc.
2.   Request that a fire extinguisher and smoke detection device be obtained. Have old newspapers, trash and flammables removed. Keep kitchen appliances free of grease.
3.   Have the telephone number of the fire department handy—that is, near the telephone.
4.   Do not leave an incapacitated client or a child alone in the home.
5.   Have a plan of escape in case of fire.
6.   Have flashlights and candles where you can find them easily in case of electrical black-out.
7.   Make sure the client's telephone is working. Know where the nearest telephone is in case the client's phone stops working (a neighbor, or a nearby pay phone). Once you reach a repair service, tell the person you are a home health caregiver and must have priority service, which they usually provide.
8.   Keep your car in good repair and make sure you have adequate gas in the tank. Understand your agency's policy regarding using your car for errands on the client's behalf or to transport a client. Plan for an alternate means of transportation, if necessary, such as a taxi or ambulance.
9.   Some regions are known for severe weather conditions that may preclude a caregiver or client leaving the house. Be prepared by

maintaining adequate food, medicine, bottled water, and home supplies. Discuss the potential problem with your supervisors, the client and the client's significant others.

10. If the client lives in a known high-crime area, check with the local police department about escort service and other means of protection for you and your client. Check with your agency on personal protection, too, such as carrying pepper spray or other devices. Make sure the client has adequate locks on windows and doors. Do not provide access to anyone you do not expect or know while caring for your client. Call the police immediately if someone tries to get in.

11. Always expect the unexpected. If a client becomes physically combative and dangerous to you, extricate yourself from contact with him or her. Call 911 and rely on the police or emergency personnel to handle the situation. Do the same for a client who suddenly decides to commit suicide or other potentially tragic act. Never be so proud as to think you alone can avert all difficulty.

Summary

- Know where you are going. Use the nurse's directions; for the most part, they are excellent.

- Carry street maps. Sometimes the visual approach works better.

- Know where the police station is. If you feel threatened, it can be a safety net.

- Know your agency's policy on "double-visit" areas.

- Keep your car in good mechanical condition. You may wish to consider a service like AAA.

- Avoid wearing flashy jewelry or carrying a handbag. Lock the bag in your trunk.

- Avoid shortcuts, and do not enter vacant buildings.

- Keep keys in your hand when approaching your car and check the back seats.

- Walk with an air of purpose and always be aware of your surroundings.

- Keep car doors locked even in what you believe to be a safe area.

Appendix: Group Discussions

The following scenarios are designed to stimulate interdisciplinary and intradisciplinary discussion and encourage critical thinking. For that reason, they are incomplete. What additional information would you seek? What would you do in each case, when action is required? Even if you are not a member of the profession in question, it still may be helpful — and memorable — for you to consider what an appropriate response might be.

Working professionals, allied-health students and home health agency non-professional personnel may benefit from group discussions on the situations they have encountered or may encounter as home caregivers.

1. A community nurse has just made her scheduled visit in a neighborhood unfamiliar to her. A young boy she doesn't know comes up to her and tells her an old man living alone in a nearby house needs help. The boy can give her no more information and he leaves. The nurse walks to the front door, which is ajar. She looks into a disorderly living room and sees an old man sitting alone in a chair, facing a TV that is on. She calls to him and he doesn't respond.

2. A home health aide is scheduled to make a first visit to an 85-year-old man who cannot walk and is deaf. The man's daughter is supposed to be present to orient the aide. When the aide arrives, the man is sitting alone on the porch and the daughter is not at home. The man seems disoriented. He greets the aide with a friendly nod and smile but mumbles incoherently in response to her questions.

3. A physical therapist arrives at a scheduled visit with a patient she has been seeing for months without negative incident. The patient is quite old but has been cooperative and responsive in the past. On this day, she tells her nurse without emotion that she would rather be alone. She refuses her treatment and tells the physical therapist to leave.

4. A young patient tells a medical social worker that his medicine makes him sick, and sometimes he spits it out when the nurse isn't looking. The social worker tells the nurse, who rebukes the patient.

On the next visit, the patient tells the social worker he won't talk to her and can't trust her because of the betrayed confidence.

5. A nurse's aide is scheduled to be in a patient's home from 3 to 11 p.m. The family members present constantly offer her food she finds unappealing. She prefers to bring her own food. The patient's mother is especially insistent and is obviously insulted when the nurse's aide refuses the food.

6. An occupational therapist is the only adult present in a teenage patient's home on a given day. The patient is locked in her bedroom with her boyfriend and doesn't answer when the OT knocks and calls her name.

7. A speech therapist has been treating a 10-year-old boy in his home. The boy insists on referring to the therapist as "baldy" when his mother is present. The therapist tells the boy that name-calling isn't polite and he doesn't like it. The boy responds that he can say whatever he wants in his house. The mother grimaces and says, "I can't control him."

8. A respiratory therapist is giving treatment to a patient. The patient's young adult sister comes into the room and takes two of the patient's narcotic pain pills, saying, "It's OK. I have a bad headache."

9. The head-injured client of an OT receives a phone call, talks for a moment, and then hands the phone to the OT. The call is from the client's employer, who wants to know how the client is doing with his therapy and when he can return to work.

10. A patient being treated for severe hypertension and stroke demands that the home health aide tell the dietitian he can't eat his food without salt.

11. An 8-year-old boy shows his physical therapist two welts on his thigh from a spanking his mother gave him. He says he made her mad. Later during the visit, the mother tells the boy he'd better "mind" or he'll get worse than that next time.

12. A nurse is treating a patient who has just been diagnosed as HIV-positive. She tells the homemaker that when she changes the linens or does any other cleaning, she should wear gloves to protect herself from contact with the patient's blood. The homemaker then says she's going to quit because she doesn't want any problems like "that."

13. During an occupational therapy session with a 90-year-old man, you discover that although he insists on shaving himself, he cuts himself each time and cannot adequately clean his face afterward.

14. You come home tired from your job as a home health aide and complain about the difficulties and low pay. Your spouse says, "I think you're crazy for working so hard. Why don't you get a different job?"

15. Today is your day off. Tomorrow promises to be an unusually stressful, complicated day that you are already dreading. How will you spend today?

16. A tuberculosis patient has a dog that sits on his bed and constantly licks him. When you approach the bed, the dog wags his tail and jumps at you to play and lick your face.

17. Two days after your patient fell as you were helping him from the bed to the bathroom, the patient's son, a lawyer, calls to discuss the incident with you. The patient says he's in pain as a result of the fall, and you have filed an incident report.

18. An elderly client repeatedly complains to the nurse's aide that she is cold and wants the windows closed, but the nurse's aide feels the room is much too warm and stuffy.

19. When you call your supervisor at the VNA to say you have the flu, she tells you you'd better go to work or she may not be able to use your services anymore. You have been working for the VNA for one year and have taken all the sick days to which you are entitled.

20. An older nurse taking care of a terminally ill cancer patient at home was informed by the home care agency that a social worker would be paying a visit the next day to talk to the patient about hospice services. The nurse had always been accustomed to handling both the physical and emotional care of her patients for the past 30 years, and she resented the "intrusion" of the social worker.

Bibliography

Chapter 1

Bowman A., Kernel C. *State and Local Government.* Boston, MA: Houghton Mifflin Co.; 1990.

Califano JA., Jr. *America's Health Care Revolution: Who Lives? Who Dies? Who Pays?* New York: Touchstone; 1986.

Fuchs VR. *Who Shall Live? Health, Economics and Social Choice.* New York: Basic Books; 1974.

Henneberger M. "Basic Care Suffers Under Medicaid in New York." New York Times, May 1, 1994, p. 1.

Hurst J, Keenan M., Minnick J. Healthcare polarities: Quality and cost. *Nursing Management* 1992;23(9).

Reagan MD. *Curing the Crisis: Options for America's Health Care.* Boulder, CO: Westview Press; 1992.

Encyclopedia of Social Work, 19th ed. Washington, DC: National Association of Social Workers, 1995.

Califano JA. *America's Health Care Revolution. Who Lives? Who Dies? Who Pays?* New York: Touchstone; 1989.

Califano JA. *Radical Surgery: What's Next For American Health Care.* New York: Times Books; 1994.

Katz MB. *In the Shadow of the Poorhouse: A Social History of Welfare in America.* New York: Basic Books; 1986.

May B. National Association for Home Care. Basic Statistics about Home Care 1994. Washington, DC. NAHC 1994.

Reagan MD. *Curing the Crisis: Options for America's Health Care.* Boulder, Co.: Westview Press Inc; 1992.

Specht H., Courtney M. *Unfaithful Angels: How Social Work Has Abandoned Its Mission.* New York: The Free Press; 1994.

Savage J. "Slums as a Common Nuisance." *The Annals of America.* Vol. 6. p. 279. The Challenge of a Continent. Chicago: Encyclopaedia Britannica; 1968.

Stevens R. *In Sickness and In Wealth: American Hospitals in the Twentieth Century.* New York: Basic Books; 1989.

Stoddard S. *The Hospice Movement: A Better Way of Caring for the Dying.* New York: Vintage Books; 1978.

Wald L. *The House on Henry Street.* New York: Holt, Rhinehart & Winston, Inc.; 1915.

Wekesser C. *Health Care in America: Opposing Viewpoints.* San Diego, Ca.: Greenhaven Press, Inc.; 1994.

Zerwekh J. Public health nursing legacy: Historical practical wisdom. *Nursing and Health Care.* 13;2:84-91.

References for Patients and Their Families

Ahronheim J., Weber, D. *Final Passages.* New York: Simon and Schuster; 1992.

Brand Covell M. *The Home Alternative to Hospitals and Nursing Homes.* New York: Rawson Associates; 1983.

Callanan M., Kelley P. *Final Gifts: Understanding the Special Awareness, Needs and Communications of the Dying.* New York: Bantam Books; 1993.

Dossey L. *Healing Words: The Power of Prayer and the Practice of Medicine.* San Francisco: HarperCollins; 1993.

DuFresne F. *Home Care: An Alternative to the Nursing Home.* Elgin, Ill.: Brethren; 1983.

Hastings D. *The Complete Guide to Home Nursing.* Woodbury, NY: Barron's Educational Series; 1986.

Jarvik L., Small G. *Parentcare.* New York: Bantam Books; 1990.

Kaiser-Sterns A. *Living Through Personal Crisis.* New York: Ballantine Books; 1984.

Kubler-Ross E. *On Death and Dying.* New York: Macmillan; 1969.

Navarra T. *Wisdom for Caregivers.* Thorofare, NJ: SLACK Inc.; 1995.

Ross S. *The Caregiver's Mission.* Plantation, FL: Distinctive Publishing Corp.; 1993.

Salamon LM. *America's Nonprofit Sector.* New York: The Foundation Center; 1992.

Siegel B. *Peace, Love and Healing.* New York: Harper and Row; 1989.

Silverstone B., Kandel Hyman H. *You and Your Aging Parent.* New York: Pantheon Books; 1989.

The U. S. Department of Health and Human Services. Landay, Eugene, ed. *The Complete Medicare Handbook.* Rocklin, CA: Prima Publishing and Communications; 1990.

Chapter 3

Andrews RG. Permanent placement of negro children through quasi-adoption. *Child Welfare.* 47:583-588.

Atchley RC. *Social Forces and Aging.* Belmont, CA: Wadsworth; 1988.

Bawer B. *A Place at the Table: The Gay Individual in American Society.* New York: Poseidon Press; 1993.

Department of Justice. Office of the Attorney General. Federal Register. July 26, 1991. 28 Cfr 36. "Nondiscriminaion on the Basis of Disability by Public Accommmodations and in Commercial Facilities: Final Rule."

Friedan B. *The Fountain of Aging.* New York: Simon and Schuster; 1993.

Fischer A, Beasley JD, Harter CL. The occurrence of the extended family at the origin of the family of procreation: A developmental approach to negro family structure. *Journal of Marriage and Family.* 30:290-300.

Geismar L, Gerhart U. Social class, ethnicity, and family functioning: Exploring some issues raised by the moynihan report. *Journal of Marriage and the Family.* 30:480-487.

Giamo B. *On the Bowery: Confronting Homelessness in America.* Iowa City, Iowa: University of Iowa Press; 1989.

Heward WL, Orlansky MD. *Exceptional Children.* Columbus, OH: Merrill Publishing Co.; 1988.

Jacobs C, Bowles D. *Ethnicity and Race: Critical Concepts in Social Work.* Silver Springs, MD: NASW Press; 1988.

Johnson Braden A. *Out of Bedlam: The Truth About Deinstitutionalization.* New York: Basic Books; 1990.

Jones TL. *The Americans with Disabilities Act: A Review of the Best Practices.* New York: AMA Membership Publications Division; 1993.

Joseph MV. Religion and social work practice. *Social Casework: The Journal of Contemprary Social Work.* Sept.1988:443-452.

Kubler-Ross E. *AIDS: The Ultimate Challenge.* New York: Macmillan; 1987.

McGoldrick M, Pearce J, Giordano J. *Ethnicity and Family Therapy.* New York: The Guilford Press; 1982.

Monette P. *On Becoming a Man: Half a Life Story.* New York: Harcourt, Brace, Jovanovich; 1992.

Murphy CB. Educating mental health professionals about gay and lesbian issues. *The Journal of Homosexuality.* 1991;22:314.

Tatara T. "Elder Abuse." *The Encyclopedia of Social Work.* 19th edition, Vol. 1, pp. 834 - 842. Washington, D.C.: National Association of Social Workers;1995.

Chapter 4

Davis CM. *Patient/Practitioner Interaction: An Experiential Manual for Developing the Art of Health Care.* Thorofare, NJ: SLACK Inc.; 1994.

Dobkin PL, Morrow G. Biopsychosocial assessment of cancer patients: Methods and suggestions. In: Dush D, Cassileth B, Turk D, eds. *Psychosocial Assessment in Terminal Care.* New York: Haworth Press, 1986.

Edelman J, Crain MB. *The Tao of Negotiation.* New York: HarperCollins; 1993.

Groves JE. Taking care of the hateful patient. *The New England Journal of Medicine.* 1978;298(16):883-887.

Haden-Elgin S. *The Gentle Art of Verbal Self-Defense.* New York: Barnes and Noble Inc.; 1993.

Rodgers C. *On Becoming a Person.* Boston: Houghton, Mifflin; 1961.

Navarra T, Lipkowitz M, Navarra J. *Therapeutic Communication: A Guide to Effective Interpersonal Skills for Health Care Professionals.* Thorofare, NJ: SLACK Inc.; 1990.

Safford F, Krell G. *Gerontology for Health Professionals: A Practice Guide.* Washington, DC: NASW Press; 1992.

Satir V. *Conjoint Family Therapy.* Palo Alto, CA: Science and Behavior Books; 1983.

Weisman A. *Coping with Cancer.* New York: McGraw-Hill; 1984.

Chapter 5

Bass D. *Caring Families: Supports and Interventions*. Silver Spring, MD: NASW Press; 1990.

Ferrer M, Navarra T. Professional boundaries: Clarifying roles and goals. *Cancer Practice*. 1994;2(4):311-312.

Holosko MJ, Taylor PA. *Social Work Practice in Health Care Settings*. Toronto: Canadian Scholar's Press; 1994.

Lubkin I. The family caregiver. In: Lubkin I, ed. *Chronic Illness: Impact and Interventions*. Boston: Jones and Bartlett; 1990.

NASW Standards for Social Work in Health Care Settings. Washington, DC.: NASW Press; 1987.

Nelson GM, Eller A, Streets D, Morse ML. *The Field of Adult Services*. Washington, DC.: NASW Press; 1995.

Silverstone B, Burack-Weiss A. The social work function in nursing homes and home care. *Gerontological Social Work Practice in Long-term Care*. New York: Haworth; 1982.

Wilson F, Neuhauser D. *Health Services in the United States*. 2nd edition. Cambridge, MA: Ballinger Publishing Co.; 1987.

Chapter 6

Zucker E. *Being a Homemaker/Home Health Aide*. Englewood Cliffs, NJ: Prentice-Hall; 1991.

Chapter 7

Dass R, Bush M. *Compassion in Action: Setting Out of The Path of Service*. New York: Bell Tower; 1992.

Freudenburger HJ, North G. The 12 stages of women's burnout. *New Woman*. Jul 1985:59-61.

Goldenberg I, Goldenberg H. *Family Therapy: An Overview.* Pacific Grove, CA: Brooks/Cole; 1985.

Kram K. *Mentoring at Work: The Role of Peer Relationships In Organizational Life.* Glenview, IL: Scott, Foresman; 1985.

Kram K, Isabella L. Mentoring alternatives: The role of peer relationships in career development. *Academy of Management Journal.* Mar 1985;28(1):110-132.

Lampert-Hill H. Point and counterpoint: Relationships in oncology care. *Journal of Psychosocial Oncology.* 1991;9(2).

Luks A, Payne P. *The Healing Power of Doing Good.* New York: Fawcett Columbine; 1991.

McElroy AM. Burnout—a review of the literature with application to cancer nursing. *Cancer Nursing.* June 1982.

Navarra T. *Wisdom for Caregivers.* Thorofare, NJ: SLACK Inc.; 1995.

Kerr ME. Theoretical base for differentiation of self in one's family of origin. In: Munson C, ed. *Family of Origin Applications in Clinical Supervision.* New York: Haworth Press; 1984.

Petersen S. Dealing with the difficult patient-family and remaining sane. *Caring.* Jan 1990:23-25.

Ray E, Nichols M, Perritt L. Model of job stress and burnout. In: Paradis L. *Stress and Burnout Among Providers Caring for the Terminally Ill and Their Families.* New York: Haworth Press; 1987.

Vachon ML. Team stress in palliative/hospice care. In: Paradis L. *Stress and Burnout Among Providers Caring for the Terminally Ill and Their Families.* New York: Haworth Press; 1987.

Yancik R. Coping with hospice work stress. *Journal of Psychosocial Oncology.* 1984;2(2):24-33.

Chapter 8

Nelson GM, Eller A, Streets D, Morse ML. *The Field of Adult Services.* Washington, DC: NASW Press; 1995.

Wilson F, Neuhauser D. *Health Services in the United States.* 2nd edition. Cambridge, MA: Ballinger Publishing Co.; 1987.

The U.S. Department of Health and Human Services. Landay E., ed. *The Complete Medicare Handbook.* Rocklin, CA: Prima Publishing and Communications; 1990.

United Way. Human Services Directory for Monmouth County. New York: Amalgamated Lithographers; 1991-1992 Edition.

Suggested Readings

Barker RL. *The Social Work Dictionary*. Silver Spring, Md: National Association of Social Workers; 1987.

Barnes M, Crutchfield C. *The Patient at Home: A Manual of Exercise Programs, Self-Help Devices, and Home Care Procedures*. Thorofare, N.J: SLACK Inc; 1984.

Bateson MC. *Composing a Life*. The Atlantic Monthly Press, New York, NY: 1989.

Beare PG, Myers JL. *Principles and Practice of Adult Health Nursing*. St. Louis, Mo: The C.V. Mosby Company; 1990.

Benson H. *The Mind/Body Effect*. New York, NY: Simon and Schuster; 1979.

Cateura LB. *Growing Up Italian*. New York, NY: William Morrow; 1987.

Clayman CB, ed. *The American Medical Association Encyclopedia of Medicine*. New york, NY: Random House; 1989.

Clinton W, Gore A. *Putting People First*. New York, NY: Times Books, Random House; 1992.

Davis CM. *Patient/Practitioner Interaction: An Experiential Manual for Developing the Art of Health Care*. Thorofare, NJ: SLACK Inc.; 1994.

Halverson RC. *No Greater Power: Perspective for Days of Pressure*. Portland, Ore: Multnomah Press; 1986.

Hermann JF, Wojtlowiak SL, Houts PS, Kahn S. *Helping People Cope: A Guide for Families Facing Cancer*. Pennsylvania Cancer Control Program, Pennsylvania Department of Health, 1988.

Jackson CL. Son, 54, charged in killings of parents, visiting nurse. The Asbury Park Press, Neptune, N.J., Nov. 18, 1995, Page 1.

Suggested Readings

Krieger D. *Accepting Your Power to Heal: The Personal Practice of Therapeutic Touch.* Santa Fe, NM: Bear & Company; 1993.

Navarra T. Cultural sensitivity: a Korean healthcare clinic. *The Nursing Spectrum.* Westbury, NY. Oct. 30, 1995.

Pear R. "Republican Governors Working With Congress to Shift Medicaid Authority to States," *The New York Times.* Sunday, April 2, 1995; National Report section, p. 20.

New York Public Health Law 2803, McKinney, 1987.

Parry W. Killer of 3 dies from own wound. The Asbury Park Press, Neptune, N.J., Nov. 21, 1995, Page One.

Roggow PA, Berg DK, Lewis MD. *The Home Rehabilitation Program Guide.* Thorofare, NJ: SLACK Inc; 1994.

Smith KS. *Caring for Your Aging Parents: A Sourcebook of Timesaving Techniques and Tips.* San Luis Obispo, Ca: American Source Books, Impact Publishers, Inc; 1994.

Stearns NM, Lauria MM, Hermann JF, Fogelberg PR. *Oncology Social Work: A Clinician's Guide.* Atlanta, GA: American Cancer Society, Inc; 1993.

Terrell TD, Andrade M, Egasse J, Munoz EM. *Dos Mundos: A Communicative Approach.* New York, NY: Random House; 1986.

Thomas CL, ed. *Taber's Cyclopedic Medical Dictionary.* Philadelphia, PA: F.A. Davis Company; 1993.

Tigges KN, Marcil WM. *Terminal and Life-Threatening Illness: An Occupational Behavior Perspective.* Thorofare, NJ: SLACK Inc; 1988.

Ulrich LT. *A Midwife's Tale: The Life of Martha Ballard, Based on Her Diary, 1785-1812.* New York, NY: Vintage Books, Random House, Inc; 1991.

Weil A. *Health and Healing.* Boston, Mass: Houghton Mifflin Company; 1988.

Williams CG. Nurse killed 'in line of duty' called vibrant, compassionate. The Asbury Park Press, Neptune, N.J., Nov. 18, 1995, Page One.

Zinn MB, Eitzen DS. *Diversity in Families*. New York, NY: HarperCollins Publishers; 1990.

Illustrated Guide to Home Health Care. Springhouse, Pa: Springhouse Corporation; 1995.

Glossary

Abnormal: deviating from the typical or acceptable (which is controversial); unusual

Abstinence: voluntary avoidance of a substance or behavior, such as abstinence from sexual activity

Abuse: improper use or treatment that may result in physical, emotional or financial harm

ACSW: Academy of Certified Social Workers

Accountability: responsibility for one's actions; being answerable to superiors and others

Accreditation: approval, acknowledgment or verification given an organization by an authoritative organization or licensing board

Acute: severe; sharp; serious

Acute care: immediate medical care of a person who is suffering from a severe condition

Addiction: compulsive need for and use of a habit-forming substance or behavior

Adult day care: program geared to non-institutionalized adults who require supervised, personal, nursing or medical care and recreational or occupational activities while their usual caregivers work or are not home

Adult protective services: human services, such as legal, medical, social, residential and custodial care, for adults who cannot take care of themselves or have no significant others to take care of them (under 1975 Title XX legislation)

Advocacy: representation of someone else's rights or cause, such as a children's advocate who participates in action taken on behalf of a child

Aftercare: the follow-up or continuing treatment and physical maintenance of clients who have been released from a hospital or institution

Agoraphobia: abnormal fear of open or public places

Alcoholism: a chronic psychological and nutritional disorder associated with excessive and compulsive drinking

Almshouse: an antiquated term for a home for the poor

Altruism: the philosophy or desire to perform services or good works for others without regard to compensation for oneself; unselfish devotion to a cause

Alzheimer's disease: a mental disease largely affecting the senior population and thought to be caused by a gradual shrinking of the frontal lobes of the brain, resulting in dementia, forgetfulness, disorientation and other symptoms that require constant supervision

Ambulatory care: medical treatment offered in doctors' offices, outpatient clinics or other facility

Glossary

Amphetamine: an addictive drug used as a stimulant; "uppers," "bennies," "speed"

Anal personality: the psychoanalytic term for an extremely fastidious or rigid person

Anemia: lack of red blood cells resulting in fatigue and other symptoms

Angina pectoris: chest pain caused by insufficient blood supply to the heart and sudden contraction of the coronary arteries

Anorexia nervosa: a life-threatening eating disorder associated with women and adolescent girls and characterized by malnutrition, excessive weight loss and the cessation of menstruation

Antidepressant medication: drugs prescribed to relieve symptoms of depression

Antipsychotic medication: drugs prescribed to lessen and/or relieve symptoms of behavior characteristic or a result of one's being out of touch with reality, eg, schizophrenic.

Antisocial: showing behavior which disrupts or threatens others

Anxiety: painful fear or uneasiness

Aphasia: absence or impairment of the ability to speak

Aphonia: inability to produce speech sounds from the larynx

Apnea: occasional or temporary failure to breathe

Assault: a physical or verbal attack which causes the victim to fear being physically harmed even if no actual physical contact is made

Assertiveness training: training a person to better express his or her true feelings

At-risk population: portions of a society comprised of people who are vulnerable or susceptible to ill or worsening health, eg, homeless mothers, the mentally ill, the frail elderly, the poor.

Atrophy: shrinking, eg, muscle atrophy as a result of inactivity or disease process

Attention deficit disorder (ADD): a disease of infancy and childhood characterized by hyperactivity, inability to pay attention and impulsivity

Autism: a syndrome, usually affecting infants and children, characterized by profound self-centeredness, language disturbances, repetitive play, rage reactions, etc.

Autonomy: independent functioning

"Bag lady": a woman who may be identified as homeless because she carries her worldly possessions in a bag

Barbiturate: a habit-forming drug that depresses the central nervous system, respiration, blood pressure and temperature

Battery: the unlawful touching of someone without that person's consent; physically injuring a person; a medical or surgical procedure performed without proper consent

Beneficence: the quality of performing good deeds or being kind

Benefits: financial help and services given by a person or organization to relieve the costs resulting from sickness, unemployment or old age

Bereavement: the state of grieving for a loss, especially of a loved one

Blamer: one who finds fault, behaves dictatorially and acts superior to others, possibly to conceal inner feelings of loneliness and a sense of failure

Blended family: chiefly, a step-family formed when two separate families are connected by marriage, eg, "The Brady Bunch"

Blocking: a temporary memory lapse

Body language: facial expressions, gestures and other physical manifestations of a person's unspoken or non-verbal feelings

Bonding: the process of becoming attached or devoted to a person, eg, mothers bonding with their infants

Boundaries: clearly defined roles and behaviors that determine a course of interpersonal interactions

Broker: one who acts on behalf of another, such as a social worker who helps a client gain access to a community service organization

Burnout: a type of depression or severe boredom resulting from excessive frustration in one's job or role

Care-and-protection proceedings: legal help for a dependent whose parent or guardian cannot or will not provide for his or her needs

Case management: the coordination of all services and helping activities for a client or clients

Catalyst: one who helps another to function differently or change, eg, a psychiatrist encouraging a client to communicate problems

Closed family: a family whose members have few, if any, relationships with people outside the family

Code of ethics: the rules, regulations, values, mission statement and principles of a professional organization

Collective responsibility: the obligation of more than one person or organization to account for a situation

Compensation: the attempt to make up for a lacking or an undesirable quality; payment for services rendered

Compulsion: mainly, a strong motivation to act a certain way or do a certain thing

Computer: one whose pattern of behavior or role is characterized by efficiency, correctness and a seeming absence of emotion

Confidentiality: the quality of being strictly private, as in the confidentiality of a client's disclosures to a therapist

Continuity of care: the coordination of services given to clients without allowing lapses or gaps to come between those services

Crisis intervention: a system of helping that is mobilized at a client's crucial time of need

Glossary

Deinstitutionalization: the release of patients or inmates from an organization that provided physical and mental care

Delirium: a state of total confusion, often induced by drugs, shock or fever, during which one may experience hallucinations, delusions, extreme anxiety and other problems

Dependency: reliance on a person for support; the excessive reliance on a substance in order to obtain a particular feeling, such as "high"

Desensitization: the diminishment or elimination of a reaction to a certain stimulus, such as allergy shots to quell the adverse effects of pollen, or treatment that results in a client's overcoming a fear or undesirable psychological reaction

Developmental disability: an impairment of growth as a result of disease or genetic disorders, eg, cerebral palsy, Down's syndrome, autism, retardation, etc.

Differentiation: see FUSION

Discharge planning: a hospital's or other organization's service designed to help patients or clients make the transition between the facility and home

Distracter: one who diverts the attention of others from the important issues, perhaps as a result of his or her feeling threatened by close relationships and acting on the desire to thwart or prevent them

Edema: generalized or local swelling in the body resulting from an accumulation of tissue fluid and frequently indicating a condition such as an infection, heart failure or kidney disease

Educator: one who teaches, provides pertinent information and offers advice

Elder abuse: the physical, mental and emotional mistreatment, neglect or exploitation of one who is aged

Enabler: one who helps another to do or achieve something, such as the ability to manage stress; also, one who believes he is helping another but is really facilitating a situation or action to the other's disadvantage or detriment

Entitlement: a certain status, such as age or condition, that allows one to receive services, goods or financial aid

Epilepsy: a seizure disorder characterized by altered states of consciousness and sometimes episodes of involuntary convulsive body movements

Ergonomics: the study of work patterns and conditions that can determine optimal efficiency and comfort on the job

Extended family: grandparents, aunts, uncles, cousins and other relatives who live with the nuclear family (parents and their children)

Facilitator: one who serves to open and coordinate communication or action among others

Family myths: distorted or altered stories or beliefs that are shared by family members without question in order to determine the members' behavior and cohesiveness

Frail elderly: aged persons who require care because they have, or may be vulnerable to, physical and emotional impairments

Friendly visitor: an antiquated term for a social worker

Fusion: the often inappropriate obscuring or uniting of two or more persons' individual identities

Gatekeeper: a leader, or one who determines the actions or communications of an organization or group

Geriatrics: one of the medical professions specializing in diseases of the elderly

Gerontology: the study of the aging process

Glaucoma: a progressive eye disease that may lead to blindness, characterized by injury to nerve cells caused by excessive fluid in and pressure of the eyeball

Goldbricking: loafing while giving the appearance of working

Grief: see BEREAVEMENT

HMO: health maintenance organization, a program that provides comprehensive health services for a fixed annual fee

Helplessness: learned passive response to the possibility of being harmed resulting from the belief that nothing or no one can help

Hierarchy of needs: Maslow's theory that people's needs range from the most essential elements of survival (food, air, water) to the need for safety, belongingness, self-respect and self-worth, to achieving one's full potential in life (self actualization)

Holistic: an attitude, practice or view geared to the entire person, ie, taking into account the biological, psychological, social and spiritual aspects

Hospice care: the provision of medical and social services to the terminally ill

Hot line: a telephone line that connects the caller immediately with a trained listener who can mobilize help or services for one in crisis

Human services: programs and services that provide assistance to those who are unable to provide for themselves

Hypertension: high blood pressure

Hypochondria: inordinate concern for, or anxiety about, one's health, usually accompanied by worry over the possibility of disease because of a symptom or symptoms

Glossary

Iatrogenic: physical or psychological illness resulting from treatment or intervention intended to be therapeutic

Identified patient (client): the person for whom some form of help is sought

Identity crisis: a profound sense of doubt over one's roles in life; confusion about behaving according to the dictates or expectations of others

Illiteracy, functional: having limited reading and writing skills

Imagery: a relaxation technique based on a person's concentration on being in a situation or place he or she finds inherently pleasurable and relaxing, such as on the beach

Implied consent: agreement on the basis of gestures, signs, actions or non-resistance, eg, appearing to willingly participate in an activity

Information and referral of a service: offered by an agency or organization to let people know of services and benefits available to them

Informed consent: permission given (usually written) by a client to health or health-related professionals that authorizes them to perform a specified procedure or intervention, based on the client's knowledge of procedures, facts, risks, etc.

Involuntary client: one who is made to receive services from professionals despite his or her own choice, eg, a prison inmate ordered to participate in psychological counseling

Kubler-Ross death stages: the emotional process leading to the acceptance of one's own death: anger, denial, bargaining, depression, acceptance

"Lady Bountiful": an obsolete (sometimes derogatory) term for social workers and volunteers who provided food, clothing and services to the needy, such as the upper-class women who served in the Civil War

Learning disability: a reading, writing or mathematical impairment or disorder in a child who is of normal or above-average intelligence

Living will: a legal document made in advance of a person's physical demise stating his or her last wishes and instructions for loved ones in the event of the person's inability to direct his own care or in the event of his death; also called an advanced directive

Long-term care: the provision of treatment and maintenance of a person who is no long able to care for him- or herself as a result of any disability, illness or injury; care may be provided in a health-care facility or in the patient's home

168

Malpractice: improper, negligent or unprofessional behavior or a failure to exercise an accepted level of skill that results in injury, loss or damage to a patient

Massage therapy: various treatments that involve relaxation and manipulation, kneading, rubbing, tapping and other techniques for therapeutic and/or rehabilitative purposes; bodywork is a general term that includes Swedish, shiatsu and other massage techniques, as well as related forms of therapeutic physical manipulation

Needs assessment: a professional evaluation of physical, emotional, social, spiritual and cultural elements lacking in a person seeking health care, in order to provide services to reestablish those elements in the person's life for the purpose of optimal well-being

Nervous breakdown: a common, non-medical term to describe various forms of mental illness that interfere with normal functioning, particularly an illness that seems to begin suddenly or that occurs as the result of a series of misfortunes or overwhelming difficulties, usually as opposed to the physical collapse of or injury to the nervous system itself

Networking: The act of creating opportunities to meet and know people with shared interests who can then lead one to others who may also be helpful; professional networking is used to find jobs, obtain educational services and locate desired sources of information

Nomadism: a condition of having no fixed dwelling place, which causes one to wander aimlessly or within a certain area, at times by choice; nomadism may be related to homelessness under certain circumstances

Nonprofit agency: an organization or group that provides services, usually humanitarian in nature, without the purpose of making a profit, that is, money over and above the group's expenditures

Nuclear family: parents and their children

Nurse practitioner: a master's-prepared nurse who is licensed to treat minor acute and chronic stable illness and, in some states so far, to prescribe medications, under the auspices of a doctor.

Open-ended question: a question that is not easily answered with a yes or no; a question that gives the opportunity for explanation or in-depth conversation

Out-patient: a person who receives medical treatment in a hospital or other facility, but who does not stay more than a day for any given treatment

Outreach: organizations or groups based in the community that provide human services or information about available services

Overloving: a term coined by Sophie Freud meaning an intense emotional attachment characterized by the desire to control the loved one "for his own good."

Paranoia: a mental disorder characterized by delusions of being persecuted; paranoid schizophrenia, on the other hand, is a psychosis that manifests in bizarre behavior, hallucinations, abnormal speech, and other symptoms that indicate a person is not in touch with reality

Paraprofessional: a person trained to perform tasks that had usually been performed by a professional, such as a paralegal or a social work associate

Parkinson's disease: progressive motor disabilities, such as shaking or tremors, muscle stiffness and impaired coordination, that usually begin in persons in their 50s and 60s

Peer group: persons of the same age group, occupation, sex, or social status

Physiatrist: a physician specializing in physical medicine, a science concerned with the diagnosis and treatment of disease and disability through radiation, heat, electricity and other physical means; physiatrists are most often affiliated with rehabilitation hospitals

Placater: one who takes on the role of peacemaker, mediator, "yes-man," subservient or penitent in order to gain approval from another person and avoid confrontation

Placebo effect: a physical result, such as relief of pain, of an individual's belief that a certain substance is working; sugar pills, often used as placebos, are identified to the individual as a potent drug before administration. A placebo may be used in conjunction with relaxation and imaging techniques to increase its effectiveness

Play therapy: toys, arts and crafts, games and other devices used by psychotherapists, social workers and others to help foster communication about a conflict or trauma when verbal communication is difficult; children and adults respond to play therapy

Pleasure principle: a Freudian theory that we come into the world seeking pleasure or gratification and avoiding pain and discomfort, and this creates a continuous desire for gratification throughout one's life; problems may arise when the gratification must at times be delayed

Post-traumatic stress disorder (PTSD): psychological and functional problems related to extraordinary stress, including natural disasters, accidents, events of war, and personal traumas, such as rape, torture or other assault or battery; persons with PTSD may have trouble working or concentrating, sleeping, experiencing typical human emotions in a normal way and may be abnormally vigilant and agitated under circumstances that would not ordinarily disturb other people

Power of attorney: a written, notarized authorization given to a person who is to act on behalf of another person who has become unable to make decisions and handle legal and financial affairs on his or her own

Practical nurse: one who completes at least 1 year of training and is licensed to perform valued but less technical nursing tasks; in some states, practical nurses are known as LPNs (licensed practical nurse), and in others they are called LVNs (licensed vocational nurse)
Prevention: action or actions that eliminate or diminish any physical, mental, social, cultural or spiritual problem or adverse condition
Professionalism: the upholding of a high standard of skills, knowledge, values and ethics of a particular profession
Prognosis: the predicted or expected outcome of a problem
Providers: professionals and organizations that perform services for a client and are then reimbursed by third-party payment organizations, such as insurance companies and federal agencies
Psychologist, clinical: one who has a master's degree or doctorate in psychology, who then counsels clients with psychosocial disorders in a private office, mental institution, hospital or mental-health facility
Psychosis: a general term for a group of severe mental disorders characterized by impaired thinking, reasoning, functioning and perception, inappropriate responses and affect, bizarre or regressive behavior, hallucinations, delusions and other symptoms

Quality assurance: a program established by an agency or organization that reviews and evaluates the effectiveness and value of its services or products

Referral: directing a client to a source of services he or she needs; referrals may be made by a professional to a specialist, agency, organization or other resource, and often include encouraging the client to accept the services and following up in order to evaluate results
Rehabilitation: the restoration of a person's ability to function and achieve an optimal physical and/or mental capacity after injury, disease, addiction, etc.
Repression: the unconscious blocking out of undesirable memories, ideas or desires in order to avoid emotional pain; according to psychodynamic theory, repression is a defense mechanism

Scapegoat: an individual or a group that is subjected to irrational hostility or blame; the term comes from the ancient Yom Kippur (Day of Atonement) ceremony, in which the people's sins are symbolically placed upon the head of a goat who is then sent into the wilderness
Seasonal affective disorder (SAD): a mood disorder characterized by depression during the months of the year that are cold and have the least amount of daylight; SAD is usually treatable by travel during winter to warm, sunny climates, or with sun lamps and other methods
Seizure disorder: See EPILEPSY

Self-actualization: the highest achievement—reaching the full potential and integrity of one's life—according to Abraham Maslow's hierarchy of needs

Senility: the deterioration of physical and/or mental functioning, such as loss of memory, as a result of old age

Shock: inadequate blood circulation to the heart caused by hemorrhage, trauma, heart attack, infection, reaction to a drug, poisoning, overdose of insulin, and other problems; symptoms of shock include extremely pale skin; cyanosis (bluish coloring) of mucous membranes, lips, fingernail beds; staring eyes; dilated pupils; weak, rapid pulse; fast, shallow breathing; urinary retention and incontinence of feces; extreme thirst; low blood pressure; possible excitement or restlessness; emergency treatment is required

Social worker: one who holds either a bachelor's, master's or doctoral degree (BSW, MSW, DSW) in social work and who is a professional member of the health care team; social workers provide counseling and psychotherapy, help clients (individuals, groups or society in general) obtain services and resources, and help communities improve social and health conditions

Soup kitchen: a designated place, such as a church hall or community room, in which food is prepared and served to the poor for a minimal charge or free of charge; charitable and religious organizations often operate soup kitchens

Stranger anxiety: fear or panic induced by the presence of unfamiliar people, including in crowds; young children may exhibit stranger anxiety

Stroke (cerebrovascular accident, CVA): a sudden blockage or impairment of blood flow to the brain that may cause body paralysis, speech and communication difficulties, sensory loss, convulsions and coma; hypertension or the clotting of blood in a blood vessel are the usual causes of stroke

Support system: a network of people, groups and organizations whose purpose is to share information, provide therapeutic communication and bolster morale among people with devastating physical or emotional problems; family members and close friends may be an individual's entire support system, but support groups have been established for victims of many diseases, addictions and other problems

Syndrome: a combination of physical symptoms, personality traits or behavior patterns that characterize a disorder or disease

Tenement: an old apartment building in a state of ill repair in which poor people live

Therapeutic Touch: a technique of rejuvenating, relaxing and rearranging an individual's energy field, which emanates from the body and projects outward, developed by Dolores Krieger, PhD, RN; a modern interpretation of ancient healing practices based on the concept that the human being is an open energy system, therapeutic touch is used to promote relaxation, reduce pain, accelerate the healing process and alleviate psychosomatic illness; this technique need not include physical contact with a patient or client; many nurses and other health professionals are becoming certified in therapeutic touch, including those at Harvard Medical School and Sloan-Kettering Memorial Hospital

Therapist: a trained professional who helps people overcome either physical or emotional disease or disability; physical therapists deal with musculoskeletal problems requiring rehabilitation; occupational therapists work with clients requiring help with activities of daily living, including work and play; there are also speech and language therapists, respiratory therapists, etc.; all are members of the health care team

Third-party payment: monetary reimbursement made by insurance companies or a government funding agency to health care workers or organizations for professional services rendered to clients

"Turf issues": difficulties or conflicts among health professionals or members of an organization concerning professional boundaries and authorization of services; for example, registered nurses offering psychological and emotional care to their clients may resent the interventions of a social worker who is also qualified to provide this type of care

Utilization review: an established process of evaluating the type and amount of an organization's or agency's services

Visiting teacher service: an education program involving school social workers who help provide tutors or educational services to students and families with special needs

Volunteer: a person who, of his or her own free will, provides needed services without charge to an individual or organization

Welfare: financial and other help provided by society to poor or disenfranchised individuals and their families

Youth service organization: an agency or organization dedicated to providing opportunities for young people to participate in sports, arts and other activities that may not ordinarily be accessible to them; examples include the YMCA, YWCA, YM/YWHA, the Boy Scouts of America, the Girl Scouts of America, etc., all organizations whose mission includes promoting social skills and moral conduct

Index

For your information

This book and many others on numerous different topics are available from SLACK Incorporated. For further information or a copy of our latest catalog, contact us at:

Professional Book Division
SLACK Incorporated
6900 Grove Road
Thorofare, NJ 08086 USA
Telephone: 1-609-848-1000
1-800-257-8290
Fax: 1-609-853-5991
E-Mail: orders@slackinc.com
WWW: http://www.slackinc.com

We accept most major credit cards and checks or money orders in US dollars drawn on a US bank. Most orders are shipped within 72 hours.

Contact us for information on recent releases, forthcoming titles, and bestsellers. If you have a comment about this title or see a need for a new book, direct your correspondence to the Editorial Director at the above address.

If you are an instructor, we can be reached at the address listed above or on the Internet at **educomps@slackinc.com** for specific needs.

Thank you for your interest and we hope you found this work beneficial.